Claudia TEIXEIRA

Factors influencing the transfer of benefits from rehabilitated language

Claudia TEIXEIRA

Factors influencing the transfer of benefits from rehabilitated language

to the non-rehabilitated language in the speech therapy of bilingual aphasic patients

ScienciaScripts

Imprint
Any brand names and product names mentioned in this book are subject to trademark, brand or patent protection and are trademarks or registered trademarks of their respective holders. The use of brand names, product names, common names, trade names, product descriptions etc. even without a particular marking in this work is in no way to be construed to mean that such names may be regarded as unrestricted in respect of trademark and brand protection legislation and could thus be used by anyone.

Cover image: www.ingimage.com

This book is a translation from the original published under ISBN 978-620-6-72193-2.

Publisher:
Sciencia Scripts
is a trademark of
Dodo Books Indian Ocean Ltd. and OmniScriptum S.R.L publishing group

120 High Road, East Finchley, London, N2 9ED, United Kingdom
Str. Armeneasca 28/1, office 1, Chisinau MD-2012, Republic of Moldova, Europe
Printed at: see last page
ISBN: 978-620-8-25332-5

Contents

Resume 2

Acknowledgements 3

I Theoretical part 5

II Method 12

III Results 15

IV Discussion 21

V Conclusion 26

Bibliographical references 27

APPENDICES 33

Resume

At a time of globalisation, the erosion of borders and migratory flows that have become more and more significant since the twentieth century, speech and language therapists are increasingly exposed to bilingual populations presenting with various cognitive and communicative disorders, including aphasia. The great variability of the resulting disorders and the diversity of bilingualism make bilingual aphasia a unique clinical entity, which cannot be reduced to a single treatment. We therefore sought to identify the factors that might be involved in the transfer of therapeutic effects from the reeducated language to the non-reeducated language. to the non-reeduced language.

To this end, a bibliometric search led to the selection, reading and qualitative analysis of twenty-six scientific articles. The status of the language treated, the typological proximity of the languages, the nature of the therapy and the nature of the elements included in the therapeutic protocol are the main factors on which it is possible to act in the hope of encouraging this transfer. Other factors such as the place of the language of the environment, the role of an interpreter in the therapy, the intensity of the rehabilitation or the state of the cognitive control circuit are discussed in more detail. These results raise important clinical implications for speech and language therapy practice.

Keywords

Aphasia; bilingualism; generalisation; inter-linguistic transfer; adult neurology; aphasiology; speech therapy; literature review

Acknowledgements

My warmest thanks to :

To Mrs Marie Faure, speech therapist, placement supervisor and dissertation director, for having supervised, trained, helped and encouraged me throughout this last year. Thank you for our many exchanges and shared moments.

To all the speech therapists who have opened their doors to me in private practice, in institutions or in hospitals. You have passed on valuable knowledge and values to me.

To Mrs Solene Hameau, speech therapist and researcher, for her bibliographical resources, her trust in me and her keen interest in my subject.

To the members of the speech therapy department's management team for accompanying me through a particular stage of my schooling.

To my future speech and language therapy colleagues and partners in adventure: Amelie, Julie, Marie and Manon, with whom I've shared these five wonderful years. You have been solid pillars throughout this course.

To my friends who have followed me and made their presence felt from near and far.

To my family, who inspired me to write this memoir.

To my parents and my sister, who believed in me and always supported me in my choices and my plans. You are my models of ambition and success.

To Clovis, for his unfailing encouragement and support over so many years.

"Language is certainly more than a simple communication tool; it is the most representative element of a culture and a civilisation, but also one of the most powerful factors in individuation and in the construction of personality". (Gatignol & Topouzkhanian, 2012)

1 Introduction

Aphasia is an acquired language disorder, which may manifest itself on the comprehension and/or expression side, occurring after cerebral damage of a vascular, traumatic, tumoral or degenerative nature (Brin, Courrier, Lederle, Masy & Kremer, 2011). Although increasingly common in speech and language therapy practice, aphasia in bilingual or polyglot patients remains little studied to date (Kopke & Prod'homme, 2009). However, with no fewer than 6912 languages recorded in over 200 countries, a large number of states admit two official languages, and current globalisation is only extending these situations (Centeno & Ansaldo, 2013). Cerebral lesions acquired in this particular patient are therefore no longer the exception but are tending to become the norm (Fabbro, 2001). For Kopke (2013), the challenges of studying bilingual aphasia are manifold. Firstly, from a theoretical point of view, recent research aims to increase scientific knowledge of both the linguistic diversity of speakers around the world and the cognitive functioning of the 'bilingual brain'. Secondly, from a clinical point of view, it is becoming essential to provide practitioners with concrete keys to understanding the assessment, recovery and language rehabilitation of these patients, whose profiles are heterogeneous and complex. This review of the literature focuses on the benefits of providing language rehabilitation in a single language to a bilingual person with aphasia (PBaA). This choice of study is explained by the fact that most rehabilitation in France is monolingual (Jaillet, 2015). More specifically, the aim is to identify the factors that enable the transfer of therapeutic benefits from the re-educated language to the non-re-educated language. The first part of our dissertation will define the concept of bilingualism and present the clinical and neurolinguistic manifestations of aphasia in the bilingual population. Recent theoretical data will then be shared on the various possible rehabilitative approaches and the issues involved in cross-linguistic transfer. In the second part, the methodology used to carry out this research and the scientific relevance of the data collected will be explained. Finally, the third and fourth parts will present the relevant results of the research and draw conclusions. Finally, the limitations of this work and future perspectives in relation to speech and language therapy practice will be discussed.

2 Aphasia in bilingual patients: clinical manifestations

2.1 Neurolinguistic semiology of bilingualism

The presence of bilingualism in the world shows that people can learn two languages without any apparent difficulty. However, this concept remains difficult to define because it covers a vast typology of speakers (Costa & Sebastian-Galles, 2014). For Grosjean (2015, p. 16), bilingualism is "the regular use of two or more languages or dialects in everyday life". It is found in all countries, whatever the age, origin, sex or socio-occupational category of its speakers. (Grosjean, 2003). Certain criteria, such as the age at which the language was acquired, the level of competence, the relative status of the language, the method and order of acquisition, commonly define the type of bilingualism of healthy subjects (Khachatryan et al., 2016). Linguist Abdelilah-Bauer (2008, p.8) believes that in reality there are 'as many ways of experiencing bilingualism as there are bilingual individuals'. It is for this reason, then, that we will talk here of bilingualism in a broader sense: not as the cohabitation of two languages alone, but sometimes of several languages in the same individual.

Knowledge and understanding of bilingual brain functioning has increased considerably in recent years, thanks to contributions from cognitive science, new imaging techniques and computational moderation (Dana-Gordon, Mazaux & N'Kaoua, 2013). Despite differing views on neural representation, it is now commonly accepted that certain linguistic processes are shared between languages (Costa & Sebastian-Galles, 2014). This conception echoes the convergence theory (Abutalebi & Green, 2007) which admits identical neural networks for the first language acquired (L1) and the second (L2). The brain structures involved are similar when bilinguals use either of their two languages, which explains why the languages activate in parallel in most contexts of use. The difference with monolingual brain function is illustrated by the need for additional neural resources. Indeed, learning a second language requires the implementation of complex cognitive processes, in particular to inhibit one language in favour of another (Abutalebi & Green, 2007; Costa & Sebastian-Galles, 2014). This shared neural network enables cross-linguistic influence at phonological, lexical and syntactic levels (Knoph, Lind & Simonsen, 2015). For example, bilinguals show non-selective lexical access, which means that even in a monolingual context, words from both languages are simultaneously active (Verreyt, De Letter, Hemelsoet, Santens & Duyck, 2013). Kroll and his team (2015) point out the multidirectional aspect of this influence: the L1 influences the speaker's other languages (L2, L3, L4, etc), which in turn influence the L1. According to Weinreich (1953, cited in Bardyn & Martin, 2012), the mental lexicon of bilinguals is organised in three different ways. Firstly, in the coordinated bilingual, i.e. when the languages have been learned separately and independently, the two 'linguistic labels' of a word in one language each correspond to their own unit of meaning. Conversely, in compound bilingualism, where the languages have been acquired in a similar fashion, the same words in the two languages converge towards a single unit of meaning. Finally, in subordinate bilingualism, where the first language has the upper hand over the second, the bilingual subject needs to go through the lexicon of his mother tongue (L1) to access the meaning of a word in his second acquired language (L2). There is ongoing debate about the exact mechanisms of language processing in bilingual aphasia (Khachatryan et al., 2016); however, the latest knowledge on the subject opens the door to possible multilingual effects caused by language rehabilitation.

2.2 Theories on language impairment and recovery patterns

As in the case of monolinguals, a cerebral lesion acquired in the dominant hemisphere for language can suddenly lead to aphasia in bilingual patients (Kohnert, 2009). The main cause is stroke, which most often affects the language-dominant cerebral hemisphere (Hernandez et al., 2001, cited in Sabadell, Tcherniack, Michalon, Kristensen & Renard, 2018). The resulting patterns of language impairment are complex and heterogeneous (Paradis, 1977), and the modes of recovery are not fixed, as a speaker's different languages constantly interact throughout the rehabilitation period (Gatignol & Topouzkhanian, 2012). In addition to the aphasic symptomatology traditionally found in the monolingual population, it is not uncommon to observe particular manifestations specific to the bilingual system.

Lorenzen and Murray (2008) refer to pathological language shifts or blends, as well as translation disorders. For Khachatryan et al (2016), these are of different kinds: the total impossibility of being able to translate, even though the ability to express oneself in each language is efficient, unconscious and involuntary translation despite the impossibility of translating voluntarily, paradoxical translation where the patient can translate in one language and express himself in another, and finally, translation without comprehension. The alternation of languages from one sentence to another or within the same sentence *(code-switching)* and translation abilities normally occur consciously in healthy bilingual speakers (Bardyn & Martin, 2012). However, in the event of an acquired brain lesion, these processes become uninhibited. They therefore occur unconsciously and may persist even when the patient has been explicitly invited to maintain the conversation in a single language (Khachatryan et al., 2016).

The clinical literature describes several phases in the recovery of language in bilingual aphasics (Fabbro, 2001). First, there is the acute phase (about four weeks after the accident), then the lesional phase (from a few weeks to 4/5 months after the accident) and finally the late phase (from a few months after the accident to the end of life). In 1977, Paradis distinguished six modes of language recovery in bilingual subjects. Firstly, it is termed 'parallel' if the two linguistic systems recover at the same rate and in equal amounts over time. If there is a more significant recovery of one language to the detriment of another, and taking into account the patient's pre-morbid linguistic abilities, this is referred to as 'differential' recovery. Recovery can also be 'selective' if only one of the languages is partially recovered by the subject. It is 'successive' if the first language recovers completely before the second begins to recover, and 'regressive' or 'antagonistic' if only one language recovers and then regresses. At the same time, the second language begins to recover. Finally, impairment is termed 'mixed' or 'blended' if the two language systems interfere with each other, resulting in a mixture of languages and significant confusion at all linguistic levels (Paradis, 1977). Research by Paradis (2000) and Fabbro (2001) found similar results, with around 60% of recuperation cases being of the 'parallel' type.

How can the diversity of recovery profiles be explained? Since the beginning of the 20th century, various authors have sought to understand the factors that can influence language recovery. Two famous theories pioneered the subject (Bardyn & Martin, 2012). In 1881, Ribot set out the following postulate in his "law of regression": the earlier a language is acquired in a person's life, the better his chances of recovery after brain damage. According to Ribot's law, the mother tongue is always the best preserved. In 1985, Pitres' law went against this hypothesis, stating that the best-recovered language would correspond to the one most used (and a fortiori the one best mastered) before the accident. Having met with great success at the time, these two laws have had the immense merit of advancing research and giving rise to other publications on the subject. Nevertheless, they remain purely theoretical at present, for the simple reason that they cannot account for all the types of recovery encountered in clinical practice (Kopke & Prod'homme, 2009). The emotional context related to each language, the age and context of acquisition, the place of the language in the environment, impairment of the cognitive system for controlling or selecting languages, the structure of the languages or cerebral localisation are all factors that have been put forward to explain recovery; but none of them has proved conclusive on its own (Bardyn & Martin, 2012). From a more current perspective, the emphasis is on the effect induced by cognitive factors (Durand, Masson-Trottier & Ansaldo, 2018). More and more studies are being carried out to analyse precisely the extent to which these factors are involved and interact. If they prove to be generalisable, future results will provide valuable insights into aphasiology.

2.3 Assessment of bilingual aphasia and language deficits

Given the serious consequences it can have, aphasia in bilinguals is a medical emergency, requiring the fastest possible multidisciplinary treatment. Once the vital prognosis has been ruled out, a more exhaustive language assessment should be carried out on the patient. This type of aphasia requires a special approach to language assessment (Hameau, 2013). Kopke and Prod'homme (2009) report that in these situations, speech and language therapy assessment of the patient is often carried out in the language of the host country only. However, a partial assessment - limited to a single language - does not provide a complete picture of the patient's language skills (Bardyn & Martin, 2012). Moreover, for several authors such as Fabbro (2001) and Paradis (1995), this is unacceptable for ethical reasons.

Paradis (2000) has suggested two reasons for reassessing the polyglot patient in all his/her languages. Firstly, when the patient no longer has access to the language of the hospital environment (host environment), it is essential to determine whether another language can be used as a means of communication. By assessing all the languages, it then becomes possible to define with a certain degree of certainty which one is the best preserved and/or the least affected. Secondly, certain deficits may only be observable in one of the two languages, and these deficits often provide valuable information about the location and extent of the acquired lesion.

Although traditional aphasia tests such as the BDAE (Boston Diagnostic Aphasia Examination, Goodglass & Kaplan, 1972) or the MT-86 (Protocole Montreal-Toulouse d'examen linguistique de l'aphasie, Nespoulous, Joanette & Lecours, 1986) have proved their effectiveness, they are still incomplete and not very sensitive to the assessment of bilingual patients in Neuro-Vascular Units (Guinel, 2013). However, Kopke and Prod'homme (2009) explain that simply translating a test from one language to another quickly comes up against phonological, lexical, morphosyntactic and even cultural biases. As a result, a number of standardised, valid and comparable assessment tools have been developed for each language. Among these, the Bilingual Aphasia Test (BAT), created by Paradis and Libben (1987), still stands out today as a major reference in multilingual assessment. A genuine battery calibrated for 65 languages, it offers a complete evaluation in three parts. Part A, which is qualitative, lists the patient's language history and multilingual skills in various situations. Part B, which is quantitative, compares phasic disorders in each language. Finally, part C estimates the patient's ability to translate from one language to another in terms of expression and comprehension (Kopke & Prod'homme, 2009). The Screening BAT, an abbreviated version of the BAT, was introduced in 2013. Currently adapted and standardised in 12 languages, it enables rapid screening for acute bilingual aphasia (Guilhem, Gomez, Prod'homme & Kopke, 2013). Whatever the test chosen by the practitioner, the patient's performance must always be interpreted in the light of his or her linguistic history (Khachatryan et al., 2016) and level of language proficiency in the two languages prior to the accident (Paradis, 2000). This valuable information is likely to explain the patterns of language alteration and the response to rehabilitation (Kiran & Iakupova, 2011).

To sum up, the aim of speech and language therapy assessment in PBaA is to highlight both the language impairments and the preserved communicative components, which will form the basis of future rehabilitation. This is followed by the implementation of a therapeutic plan and patient follow-up (Chomel-Guillaume, Leloup & Bernard, 2010).

3 Rehabilitation of bilingual aphasia and the challenges of inter-linguistic transfer

3.1 Different types of rehabilitation possible

Initiated early and intensively (Sabadell et al., 2018), speech and language therapy for PBaA is just as particular and individualised as the language assessment process. As early as 1986, Kraetschmer highlighted an important issue: the therapist must give priority to the language that will bring out the most progress in the patient. But how do you choose? Which language should be re-educated" (Chomel-Guillaume et al., 2010, p. 97), "Should one language be treated preferentially? If so, which one? Or should we encourage the involvement of both languages? (Mung & Claivaz, 2016, p. 29). Unlike the more classic cases of monolingual aphasia, intervention in bilingual aphasia has never been justified: either by a theoretical approach or by a model of language production (Ansaldo, Saidi & Ruiz, 2010). Sabadell et al (2018) propose three possible rehabilitation options: rehabilitation of both languages, carried out at the same time or one after the other, or selective rehabilitation, i.e. specific to one language. Ansaldo, Saidi and Ruiz (2010, cited in Durand et al., 2018, p. 42) explained the value of reeducating both languages with the following argument: "if the bilingual language system is not two language systems in one, but a complex integration of two languages into one system, therapy with a PBaA should be done in both languages." Yet monolingual rehabilitation currently seems to be the most widely used in French speech and language therapy clinical practice (Jaillet, 2015). Radman, Spierer, Laganaro, Annoni and Colombo (2016) explain this for three reasons. Firstly, dual therapy can cognitively overload the patient and consequently induce involuntary and pathological linguistic productions (Edmonds & Kiran, 2006; Fabbro, 2001; Kiran, Sandberg, Gray, Ascenso & Kester, 2013; Mazaux, Pradat-Diehl & Brun, 2007), or even prevent the recovery of one of the languages (Faroqi-Shah, Frymark, Mullen & Wang, 2010). Secondly, bilingual rehabilitation is often limited for logistical and practical reasons. Indeed, the lack of time allocated to such rehabilitation (Fabbro, 2001) and the shortage of bilingual therapists (Kopke, 2013) hinder its successful implementation. Thirdly, if we assume that bilinguals share common lexical and morphosyntactic processing (Gollan, Montoya, Fennema-Notestine & Morris, 2005), then monolingual therapy would be the most appropriate way of improving both languages, particularly if the effects of treatment in the first language generalise to the second (Faroqi-Shah et al., 2010; Kohnert, 2009). Bilingual aphasic patients are therefore usually cared for in the language mastered by nursing staff and speech and language therapists. For a large number of patients with an immigrant background, this is their L2, corresponding to their second acquired language (Laganaro, 2014). This choice of treatment has proved effective (Laganaro, 2014) and does not seem to hinder bilingual recovery (Kohnert, 2009). In all cases, rehabilitation must always aim to achieve the most functional communication possible and be based on the patient's preserved skills, whatever language they speak (Ansaldo et al., 2010). Taking into account the patient's relationship with the language, their living environment, and their personal, family and socio-professional needs are all important factors which the speech and language therapist must take into account (Bardyn & Martin, 2012).

3.2 Factors influencing inter-linguistic transfer

Parallel to this functional vision of rehabilitation, the question of the transfer of language benefits between languages has emerged since the 2000s (Knoph et al., 2015). Ansaldo and his team (2010, p. 310) define Inter-Linguistic Transfer (ILT) as "the reciprocal influence that one language exerts on another". This definition reveals the notion of 'generalisation', i.e. can the linguistic progress achieved through rehabilitation in one language have an effect on a second language? In other words, can we expect a language to improve indirectly, without first having been reeducated? If most current studies choose to introduce only one language into rehabilitation, it is because they aim to induce TIL more easily (Faroqi-Shah et al., 2010; Kohnert, 2009) and to understand the underlying factors that may predict it (Conner et al., 2018). In the field, TIL is useful because bilingual individuals need to be able to use their two (or more) languages in everyday activities; it therefore seems necessary, if not essential, to create all the conditions conducive to the recovery and/or use of these languages (Kohnert, 2009).

A recent article by Durand, Masson-Trottier and Ansaldo (2018) presents the various factors with a potential for cross-linguistic transfer. First of all, the typological proximity between two languages, i.e. their degree of similarity, could come into play. Spanish and Catalan, which are close languages, as opposed to English and Chinese, which are distant languages (Conner et al., 2018), will, for example, have more lexical, morphological and semantic representations in common (Kopke, 2013). This variable can be explained by the *Multilingual* Processing Model (De Bot, 2004). Indeed, when a speaker chooses to speak in a language, this generates the activation of elements specific to that language, but also elements common to other languages. Secondly, the type of elements used in therapeutic protocols is not a trivial criterion. Ansaldo and Saidi (2014) distinguish between cognate words, which are very similar in sound and visual form and have the same meaning, such as '*tiger*' and 'tigre'; homophones, which are pronounced the same but have a different meaning, such as '*bell*' and 'belle'; and non-cognate words, which differ in phonological form and meaning, such as '*butterfly*' and 'papillon'. Goral, Rosas, Conner, Maul and Obler (2012, p. 545) specify that cognates are "two translation equivalents that share three consecutive sounds (e.g. lune - *luna*) or three consonants (e.g. curtain - *cortina*)". According to Costa, Santesteban and Cano (2005), bilinguals are faster at recognising, translating or producing this type of word because of their strong lexical link.

Thirdly, Durand, Masson-Trottier and Ansaldo (2018) highlight the status of the language treated, i.e. the patient's language competence, correlated with the direction of the transfer. According to Hameau and Kopke (2015), the TIL differs according to whether the language reacquired is major, i.e. the language that performed best before the accident, or minor, i.e. the language that performed least well. According to the *Revised Hierarchical Model (RHM*, Kroll & Stewart, 1994), "connections are stronger between the L1-specific lexicon and concepts (which are shared between the bilingual's two languages) than between the L2-specific lexicon and concepts" (Hameau, 2013, p. 89). The L1 lexicon is also more important than the L2 lexicon and lexical links are more robust from L2 to L1 than vice versa (Mung & Claivaz, 2016). The *Selection by Proficiency* (*SbP)* model *(*Schwieter & Sunderman, 2009) goes further by stating that bilinguals with low L2 proficiency (or 'non-equilibrium bilinguals') generally produce their words from lexical borrowings from the L1. In this case, processes of selection of the target word and inhibition of other words are involved.

In contrast, high-level bilinguals in their two languages (or 'balanced bilinguals') have a well-separated lexicon in L1 and L2, facilitating activation of the chosen word (Mung & Claivaz, 2016). The two schematic models are explained in Appendix A. Fourthly, the nature of the therapy (for example, reeducating the patient through semantic or phonological therapy), would not allow the same potential for TIL (Durand et al., 2018). In general, treatments targeting underlying processes common to two languages, such as semantic organisation, would be more effective than treatments focusing on language-specific structures, such as the lexicon (Conner et al., 2018).

Finally, the presence of an interpreter with the speech and language therapist during rehabilitation (Croft, Marshall, Pring, & Hardwick, 2010; Durand et al, 2018), the use of the language of the environment at the time of treatment (Goral, Rosas, Conner, Maul & Obler, 2012; Knoph et al., 2015), the degree of intensity of therapy (Radman et al., 2016) and the state of the cognitive control circuit (Ansaldo et al., 2010; Durand et al., 2018). These factors, which are less frequently described, require further publication to confirm their validity.

In the literature, several authors agree that there is a transfer from the re-educated language to the non-re-educated language, but not systematically (Faroqi- Shah et al., 2010; Kohnert, 2009; Laganaro, 2014). Debates remain open as to the influence of all the above-mentioned factors. We will attempt to analyse them in more detail in the next section.

4   Objectives of the literature review

Our literature review will attempt to identify and evaluate studies that have measured cross-linguistic transfer in the context of monolingual rehabilitation in bilinguals with aphasia. Our main objective is to identify and report on the various factors influencing the generalisation of learning. To this end, the present work will highlight important recent scientific advances, while presenting clinically relevant information for rehabilitation. At present, there is still no consensus on the choice of rehabilitation for bilinguals. This is why this issue is part of the 'Evidence-Based Practice' (EBP) movement, which uses objective research data to help clinicians make the best therapeutic choice for their patients.

II Method

The literature search was carried out from September 2018 to January 2019. A systematic review of the literature was then carried out using the precise methodology of Zaugg, Savoldelli, Sabatier and Durieux (2014), detailed below.

1 Definition of the research question and eligibility criteria

1.1 Context of the study and research question

In a globalised world, speech and language therapists are increasingly exposed to bilingual populations with various cognitive and communicative disorders, including aphasia. The focus of rehabilitation with bilingual patients is a real challenge; the aim is to encourage as much language production as possible in order to achieve the most functional communication possible. The research question was constructed on the basis of this theoretical context. In the present study, the aim is to examine the value of monolingual speech therapy in the treatment of bilingual aphasia in adults, and to look more closely at the factors that may influence the transfer of benefits from the re-educated language to the non-re-educated language. This research question, the starting point for an iterative and recursive approach, made it possible to establish strict criteria with a view to defining the scope of the research.

1.2 Eligibility criteria

The articles selected had to meet certain inclusion criteria in three areas: type of study, type of population studied and type of intervention carried out. More specifically, in the area of study type, the criteria were as follows: 1)   publication between 2000 and 2018,   2) valid   publication source
scientifically recognised by peers, 3) written in English, French or Portuguese, 4) precise scientific methodological framework for research articles according to the procedure: summary / method / results / discussion / conclusion, 5) single case study, multiple case study, meta-analysis, literature review or grey literature. With regard to the type of population studied, all the articles selected met the following criteria: 1) adult patient, 2) bilingual or multilingual patient, 3) patient with aphasia due to diagnosed cerebrolesion. Finally, concerning the intervention aspect, our requirements related to : 1) accuracy of rehabilitation: type and frequency of care, choice of language used in treatment, areas targeted by treatment, 2) accuracy of direct and indirect results of treatment: evaluation of therapeutic progress and inter-linguistic transfer (ILT). The linguistic typology and geographical region covered by the studies were not used as selection criteria, at the risk of excluding too many resources and biasing the results.

2 Implementation of the research strategy and selection of studies

2.1 Sources of bibliographical data

The literature was collected in French and English from several sources, to make the search as exhaustive as possible. The types of publications searched were experimental case studies (single and multiple), literature reviews and meta-analyses. In September 2018, a first advanced search on the Google Scholar search engine allowed us to probe the depth of results on our topic and the suitability of keywords. 643 results appeared over the time period 2000-2018, including the English keywords 'aphasia', 'bilingualism', 'cross-linguistic transfer' and excluding the concept 'children'. The literature was progressively searched and obtained via scientific and medical databases (PubMed, ScienceDirect, LiSSa), academic databases (Sudoc) and speech and language therapy databases (ASHA). In addition, a smaller number of references were found by scanning bibliographies from the DRTO (Dossier de Reflexion Thematique en Orthophonie) or from previously read articles. Finally, third parties (dissertation director, classmate, speech therapist-researcher) pointed us to additional resources, available on HAL (Hyper Articles en Ligne), ResearchGate and Taylor and Francis Online, among others. The general characteristics of the various databases are presented in Appendix B.

2.2 Database interrogation strategies and study selection

The first stage of the bibliographic dissertation was to translate the research question into keywords. Le portail HeTOP *(Health Terminology/Ontology Portal)* veritable outil de reference pour la terminologie des concepts en sante, nous a aide a definir les principaux termes MESH *(MEdical Subject Headings)* :   « aphasia »
(aphasia), *'rehabilitation'* (reeducation) and *'multilingualism'* (multilingualism). These concept words combined with Boolean operators (AND, OR, NOT) and other key words or expressions such as 'bilingualism', 'cross-linguistic *transfer*' and '*children*' resulted in an initial search equation tested on PubMed. A simple or advanced search was carried out depending on the database. Filters were used for the date of publication of articles (2000-2018) and the type of article (research articles). Details of the keywords, the search methods used for each database and the results obtained are available in Appendix C. In total, this systematic literature review includes twenty-six documents and more precisely thirteen single case studies, six literature reviews, five multiple case studies, one retrospective discussion of a single case study and one article composed of a literature review and a single case study.

3   Data extraction

From September 2018 to March 2019, the search history was documented and implemented in a *sourcing* table including the article search date, title, author(s), publication year, publication source and associated disciplinary sector, source interrogation strategy, source reliability, type of study and publication language. Finally, in order to be able to find these references easily, the keywords of the article, the URL of the document and the DOI *(Digital Object Identifier)* have been annotated. At the same time, a reading grid was completed after reading each article previously selected. The information gathered was allocated to different headings in relation to the original question. The first column (author / year / source / title of study / objectives) presents the study as a whole. The second column focuses specifically on the methodology, presenting the population studied and the intervention protocol used. Finally, the third and last column presents the direct and indirect results of the intervention, then draws the conclusions of the study and any limitations. This detailed reading grid made it possible to provide all the data required for their analysis. An example of these two documents is available in appendices D and E. Finally, the collection and management of the results were facilitated by the use of Zotero, a bibliographic reference management software. The data collection was consolidated as the research progressed. Once retrieved, the articles were deduplicated, classified, missing fields completed and their notation harmonised.

4 Assessment of the methodological quality of studies
4.1 Single and multiple case studies
The Santiago-Delefosse (2004) grid presented in Appendix F was used to qualitatively re-evaluate the single and multiple case studies. Each article was individually analysed and rated according to 22 criteria. The score obtained was then translated into a percentage of methodological quality. The average of the nineteen case studies selected was 80%. The study by Croft, Marshall, Pring and Hardwick (2010) achieved the highest percentage of quality, scoring 100%. In contrast, the studies by Knoph (2013) and Goral, Levy and Kastl (2007) scored only 32% and 41% respectively. With very little in the way of theoretical references and methodological explanations, the latter studies are more akin to the princeps versions or short summaries, rather than the original studies. Despite their low percentages, these two succinct studies have been retained in the systematic literature review, in the absence of their original, more exhaustive versions.

4.2 Literature reviews
Firstly, the reading of the literature reviews was facilitated by the PRISMA collective grid (Moher, Liberati, Tetzlaff, Altman & the PRISMA Group, 2009). Secondly, their methodological quality was analysed in accordance with the revised R-AMSTAR list (Kung et al., 2010), adapted from the initial AMSTAR grid (Shea et al., 2007). Eleven questions each score 0 to 4 points on the study selection process, the characteristics of the studies selected, the quality assessment of the studies and the methodology used for the statistical analysis (Zaugg et al., 2014). Following the analysis, a final score out of 44 points and a percentage corresponding to this score were assigned. The results of our analyses, reproduced in Appendix G, show an average of 45% methodological quality for the seven resources. The lowest quality review was Lorenzen and Murray (2008) with 32%. In contrast, Faroqi-Shah et al (2010) obtained a rate of 75%. Despite a general quality average of less than 50%, all the literature reviews analysed were retained in the final bibliometrics for two reasons. Firstly, they all contained at least one article corresponding to our inclusion criteria and able to provide significant information on our research question. Secondly, they all provided a relevant clinical perspective, or even recommendations for good practice in the treatment of bilingual aphasics.

1 Results of the systematic search

By adding together the resources obtained from the databases (n= 177) and from other sources (n= 11), a total of 188 studies were identified. After removing duplicates (n= 10), manual analysis began on 178 documents. An initial selection by reading abstracts, analysing keywords and applying search criteria resulted in the elimination of 148 articles. The reasons for exclusion were as follows: absence of bilingual patients, absence of diagnosed aphasia, absence of speech therapy mentioned, absence of inter-linguistic transfer mentioned, or a combination of all these reasons. A second selection was made on the basis of a full reading of the thirty remaining eligible articles. In the end, twenty-six papers were included in the literature review. A flow chart, documented in Appendix H, summarises the main stages of the selection process.

2 Characteristics of the studies

The design of these twenty-six studies is heterogeneous, with thirteen single case studies (50%), six literature reviews (23%), five multiple case studies (19%), two miscellaneous articles (8%) identified as a discussion of a single case study and one mixed article combining a theoretical literature review and a single case study. In the period 2000-2018, six studies (23%) were published before 2009 and twenty studies (77%) afterwards, showing a growing interest in the subject. Almost all of the selected publications (92%) were written and published in English, with only 8% in French. No references in Portuguese were obtained. All the studies listed were published in journals or newspapers recognised by the scientific community. No grey literature resources, such as dissertations, theses or conference reports, specifically targeted our subject. In addition, secondary references, known as second-hand references, were obtained through literature reviews. By deleting studies already analysed individually or which could not be retrieved from databases and publications prior to 2000, we arrive at a total of thirty eligible studies for our subject. Once the duplicates had been eliminated, twelve experimental studies were finally exploitable in this way (see Appendix I).

3 Characteristics of participants

Adults with bilingual or multilingual aphasia represented the study population. Taking into account the single and multiple case studies plus the twelve other studies extracted from the literature reviews, the age distribution ranged from 17 years for one of the subjects in Conner et al. (2018) to 88 years in the studies by Kiran, Grasemann, Sandberg and Miikkulainen (2013) and Kiran, Sandberg et al. (2013). The average age is 57 years and 5 months and the distribution of subjects is homogeneous, with 29 women and 25 men. There is a wide diversity of languages studied, including Romance languages (French, Spanish, Catalan, Italian, Friulian), Celtic (Welsh), Germanic (English, German, Swiss German, Norwegian, Dutch, Russian, Slovenian, Flemish), Indo-Iranian (Persian, Bengali), Sino-Tibetan (Chinese), Chamito-Semitic (Arabic, Hebrew) and Japanese (EOLE, 2003). Cases of English-Spanish bilingualism are the most frequently cited.

4 Characteristics of interventions

The experimental protocols began between six months (Kiran, Grasemann et al.,

2013) and eight years (Faroqi-Shah et al., 2010) after the patient's brain injury. Before each speech therapy intervention, all the patient's languages were systematically assessed. The use of tests derived from speech therapy batteries, calibrated with tasks assessing expression and comprehension, or self-assessment questionnaires, provided an insight into the patient's linguistic skills and, a fortiori, his aphasiological profile. The nature of the speech therapy provided varied considerably between studies. It could be phonological therapy, general semantic therapy or more specific semantic therapy (*SFA - Semantic Feature Analysis,* Boyle & Coehlo, 1995), and very frequently a combination of the two. Some forms of rehabilitation have targeted a particular area, such as anomia (*CIAT - Constraint Induced Aphasia Therapy,* Pulvermuller et al. 2001; *SBTT - Switch Back Through Translation*, Ansaldo et al., 2010), fluency (*ORLA - Oral Reading for Language in Aphasia*, Cherney, 2004), reading or cognitive words. Finally, from a more ecological perspective, some authors have opted for a comprehensive approach, with a cognitive or communicative focus (*PACE - Promoting Aphasics' Communicative Effectiveness*, Davis & Wilcox, 1981). Practised intensively, with several sessions per week, rehabilitation lasted from two weeks (Marangolo, Rizzi, Peran, Piras & Sabatini, 2009) to six months (Filiputti, Tavano, Vorano, De Luca & Fabbro, 2002, cited in Kohnert, 2009). It could also be stopped based on a criterion of the subject's effectiveness; for example, until the patient achieved 80% accuracy on the items targeted by the protocol. The therapy was carried out in one of the languages mastered by the patient, i.e. their mother tongue (L1) or one of their other languages (L2, L3 or L4). In order to determine the linguistic influence and to cross-check the results, it is not unusual for several languages to have been treated successively in the same patient, or for several patients in the same study to have been assessed in different languages. All studies reported the presence of at least one bilingual or multilingual speech and language therapist performing pre-treatment language assessment, speech and language rehabilitation and post-treatment language assessment. Only Croft et al (2010) reported the participation of several Bengali-speaking assistants under the supervision of the principal SLT, who was himself the study investigator.

5   Results of interventions

5.1 Studies demonstrating the absence of generalisation to the untreated language

An absent or non-significant generalisation of the benefits of the re-educated language to the non-re-educated language has been reported in several studies. Following therapy administered in L2 (German / English / French) to each of their respective participants, Meinzer, Obleser, Flaisch, Eulitz and Rockstroh (2007), Miller Amberber (2012) and Radman et al. (2016) report effects limited solely to the language treated. Thus, patients' performance in L1 (respectively: French/French/Persian) did not improve. Ansaldo et al (2010) in turn demonstrated a notable absence of improvement in Spanish, the second language (L2), after treatment in English, the subject's mother tongue (L1). Some authors carried out successive rehabilitation in several languages: in Spanish and then in English for the participant in Galvez and Hinckley (2003), in Swiss-German and then in French for the participant in Mung and Claivaz (2016). After each session, both patients made progress only in the language targeted by the therapy, which attests to direct effects of the treatment rather than indirect effects. In other cases, the absence of TIL was compounded by the pejoration of one of the patient's languages. In a 56-year-old patient with parallel aphasia in both languages, performance in Spanish (L1) on the BAT regressed at the same time as it improved in Italian (L2), the language of treatment (Abutalebi, Rosa, Tettamanti, Green & Cappa, 2009). Similarly, performance in English (L2) was negatively affected by treatment in Persian (L1), compared with initial performance in a trilingual Persian-German-English aphasic patient (Goral, Naghibolhosseini & Conner, 2013). In some multiple case studies, the absence of TIL is notable for the majority of participants. For example, in a study by Kiran and Roberts (2010) of two French (L1)-English (L2) bilinguals and two Spanish (L1)-English (L2) bilinguals, no L2-to-L1 TIL occurred for three participants. In a large sample of 17 native Spanish and English second language early bilinguals with aphasia secondary to stroke, TIL was far from the majority: it occurred in only three (Kiran, Grasemann et al., 2013) and six patients (Kiran, Sandberg et al. (2013).

5.2 Studies demonstrating the presence of generalisation to the unprocessed language

The transfer of knowledge to the untreated language is rarely total. Rather, it is partial, depending on a number of distinct factors, which we will present below.

5.2.1 Generalisation according to language status

Edmonds and Kiran (2006) report that L1 ■> L2 or L2 ■> L1 transfers are not equivalent. They therefore wished to study inter-linguistic generalisation patterns in three English-Spanish bilinguals with aphasia. The first patient was equally proficient in both languages before the aphasia. After semantic processing in Spanish, cross-linguistic generalisation was observed. The second and third participants, both of whom had a better command of English than Spanish, showed a TIL in English after semantic rehabilitation in Spanish. Interestingly, the second participant also underwent semantic processing in her major language (English), which did not result in generalisation to her minor language (Spanish). Although different, these patterns of results are each time coherent with the level of pre-morbid language competence of each participant. Several studies confirm this trend. A 57-year-old late bilingual who received treatment in Hebrew (L2) improved in Hebrew and even more so in Russian, his mother tongue and major language (Gil & Goral, 2004). After proposing semantic therapy in the weaker language (L2 - English), Kiran and Iakupova (2011) observed an improvement in the items trained in the stronger language, which had not been directly trained (L1 - Russian). Knoph (2010) reports that generalisation occurred in Arabic, the most competent language (L1), following semantic and phonological therapy in English (L2). The quadrilingual patient of Goral, Rosas, Conner, Maul and Obler (2012) showed no TIL from Spanish, his high proficiency language, to German, English or French, his three lowest proficiency languages. Following on from the work of Edmonds and Kiran (2006) concerning the link between balanced bilingualism and TIL, Marangolo et al (2009) offered a patient with high proficiency in Flemish and Italian a therapy to improve her lack of the word. After two weeks of rehabilitation in Italian, the results showed a significant increase in performance on a naming task in L2 and L1. Kurland and Falcon (2011) found the same thing: their highly educated patient, proficient in Spanish (L1) and French (L2), improved in both languages after three phases of treatment (Spanish, English and mixed). A very recent study (Conner et al., 2018) analysed the interaction between seven languages in a single patient. This 65-year-old man benefited from a general protocol to improve oral production, delivered in Dutch, his mother tongue. After 40 hours of therapy, he showed significant generalisation in German, French, English and Italian, the four languages in which he had the best command prior to his stroke; and much less generalisation in Spanish and Norwegian, his two languages of lower command. On the contrary, other studies have shown cases of TIL occurring according to post-morbid linguistic dominance. The three cases of TIL reported by Croft et al (2010) occurred after processing from the more proficient language (L1 - Bengali) to the less proficient language (L2 - English) following stroke.

In speakers of more than two languages, the TIL may remain uncertain or even unpredictable. Filiputti et al (2002) report the case of a quadrilingual man with Wernicke's aphasia. After six months' treatment in Italian (L2), his BAT scores increased in Friulian (L3) and English (L4). However, TIL did not occur in Slovenian (L1). The re-test phase four years later showed that the gains in L2, L3 and L4 were maintained and that L1 showed a pejoration. Similarly, a generalization of gains from L2 to L3, but not from L2 to L1, was reported in a trilingual Hebrew-English-French patient receiving double treatment in English. The first targeted grammatical constructions and the second anomia (Goral et al., 2007). Other cases of partial transfer of the same type have been reported by Miertsch, Meisel and Isel (2009), Goral et al. (2012), Knoph (2013) and Knoph et al. (2015).

In each case, the results show a possible transfer between the second languages (L2 to L3, L3 to L2 and L4, L4 to L2 and L3, for example), but limited or even non-existent in the direction of the mother tongue (L1).

5.2.2 Generalisation according to the typological proximity of languages

Some results show a clear advantage of TIL between languages of the same family in patients speaking three or more languages. This is the case between English and French, as opposed to Hebrew (Goral et al., 2007), between Spanish and Catalan, as opposed to Chinese (Dieguez-Vide, Gich-Fulla, Puig-Alcantara, Sanchez-Benavides, & Pena-Casanova, 2012), between English and French, as opposed to German (Miertsch et al., 2009) or between Norwegian, German and English, as opposed to Japanese (Knoph, 2013; Knoph et al., 2015). Similarly, Kohnert (2004) and Kiran and Roberts (2010) link the success of TIL between English and Spanish and between French and Spanish to the proximity of the languages involved.

Contradictory results, such as those of Conner et al. (2018), have shown a much more pregnant TIL between dissimilar languages (from Dutch to French, for example), and less convincing between typologically close languages (from Dutch to German, for example). TIL has also been found between very different language pairs, such as Italian and Flemish (Marangolo et al., 2009), Arabic and English (Knoph, 2010) or Bengali and English (Croft et al., 2010).

5.2.3 Generalisation according to therapeutic approach

As mentioned above, speech therapy treatment for aphasia can be carried out using different approaches. A comparison of the results obtained between two very different treatments was reported by Croft et al. (2010). Five participants first underwent semantic treatment (semantic association tasks, functional questions, evocation on definitions, SFA therapy), then phonological treatment (repetition tasks on target items in the presence of images, phonological indigenization, rhythm judgement, syllable counting, initial phoneme judgement) over a total duration of 10 hours, in English and Bengali. The post-test naming test showed an absence of TIL after phonological indigenization, whereas semantic indigenization elicited TIL for three out of five participants. Knoph et al (2015) found partial generalisation of verbs, syntactic and discourse features in two unprocessed languages after semantic processing with SFA. In general, many authors have noted the possibility of transfer to the non-repeated language after an intervention that includes a semantic approach in part or in full (Ansaldo & Saidi, 2014; Edmonds & Kiran, 2006; Goral et al, 2012; Hameau & Kopke, 2015; Kiran, Grasemann, et al., 2013; Kiran & Iakupova, 2011; Kiran & Roberts, 2010; Kiran, Sandberg, et al., 2013; Knoph, 2013; Kohnert, 2004).

In their review of the literature, Lorenzen and Murray (2008) report conclusive TIL results when the treatment targets linguistic representations shared between languages. This was the case with a bilingual patient who benefited from a rehabilitation treatment for alexia (Laganaro & Overton Venet, 2001). The transfer from Spanish (L1) to English (L2) was achieved for common processes - such as the lexical decision task -, whereas specific processes - such as reading aloud words and non-words - only resulted in benefits limited to the language treated (Kohnert, 2009; Laganaro, 2014). Similarly, Conner et al (2018) used ORLA therapy targeting global fluency; and as they had hoped, progress in the treated language was partially transferred to other languages.

5.2.4 Generalisation according to the type of elements used in therapy

In 2004, Kohnert set out to determine the conditions for the transfer of inter-linguistic gains in a 67-year-old man suffering from severe transcortical motor aphasia in his two languages. A two-week language protocol was administered equally in Spanish and English. The aim was to name twenty images consisting of ten cognate words and ten non-cognate words. The treatment, conducted in Spanish (L1), showed a TIL in English (L2), manifesting itself only for images containing cognate words. An earlier study (Lalor & Kirsner, 2001) reached similar conclusions after observing much better performance for cognates in naming and lexical decision tasks in Italian and English. The advantage of cognates has been demonstrated by other authors. For example, a highly proficient bilingual speaker followed a lexical protocol and showed improvement for untreated English words translated from treated Welsh cognate words. No improvement was found for unprocessed English words translated from processed non-cognate Welsh words (Hughes, Roberts & Tainturier, 2012). In naming tasks presented to another multilingual speaker, cognate words in the processed language were more often correct than incorrect in the unprocessed languages, compared to non-cognate words in the processed language (Goral et al., 2012). However, other studies show more contrasting and even contradictory results. For example, Kurland and Falcon (2011) tested the effects of a three-phase intensive naming therapy (Spanish, English and mixed) on the intra- and inter-linguistic generalisation of cognate and non-cognate words in a woman with chronic and severe expressive aphasia. They concluded that on average, in all training conditions, naming accuracy was superior for non-cognate words compared with cognate words. This inhibition of cognates occurred bidirectionally between L1 and

L2. Finally, from a more neutral perspective, Hameau and Kopke (2015) found no significant difference between cognate and non-cognate words partially transferred from French (L3) to German (L1) after three weeks of intensive lexico-semantic treatment.

5.2.5 Generalisation according to other factors

The question of the effects of therapy with a mediator acting as an interpreter between clinician and patient has been frequently raised. For Croft et al (2010), the positive results in Bengali show that rehabilitation by a third party supervised by a speech therapist is effective. Faroqi-Shah et al (2010) do not provide sufficiently clear conclusions on this issue. On the other hand, few authors have studied the influence of environmental language on TIL. In a study conducted in New York with a polyglot aphasic patient, Goral et al (2012) reported major direct improvements after the English treatment phase, compared with minor changes following the Spanish treatment phase. They also attributed the partial TIL in French and German to the linguistic environment, without providing any further explanation. Knoph et al (2015) found no relationship between therapy in the language of the patient's environment and partial TIL in the other three languages. With regard to the frequency of rehabilitation, Marangolo and his team (2009) reported robust TIL after intensive therapy lasting two hours a day, five days a week for a fortnight. Finally, damage to the cognitive control circuit prevented the generalisation of skills from Spanish to English in the patient of Ansaldo et al. (2010). What is more, adverse linguistic consequences emerged, such as unintentional linguistic blends and erroneous translations, which impeded communication.

IV Discussion

The aim of this dissertation was to examine the indirect effects of monolingual speech therapy on a bilingual aphasic. More specifically, the aim was to identify the various factors influencing the generalisation of learning from the treated language to the untreated language. A systematic literature search led to the selection of twenty-six documents. A meticulous analysis of each study enabled us to identify the factors that promote or inhibit inter-linguistic transfer (ILT). The results proving the occurrence of TIL will be presented and discussed, in relation to the theoretical elements evoked in the first part. Finally, the limitations of this literature review and clinical perspectives for speech and language therapy practice will be presented.

1 Discussion of the main results

1.1 Influence of the status of the language

Edmonds and Kiran (2006) were the first to demonstrate different cases of cross-linguistic generalisation, but these were individually dependent on their pre-morbid language skills. Their initial findings are consistent with the RHM model (Kroll & Stewart, 1994), which shows stronger links between the semantic conceptual system and the most proficient language (generally L1) than between the conceptual system and the least proficient language (generally L2). On the other hand, if we return to the principle of linguistic dependence in non-equilibrium bilinguals (Schwieter & Sunderman, 2009), a minor language is accessed through a major language. Thus, re-educating the weaker language strengthens the pre-existing links between it and the stronger language, and ultimately improves both languages (Kiran & Iakupova, 2011). On the other hand, treatment is more easily conducive to TIL in high-level balanced bilinguals, regardless of the language targeted by rehabilitation (Edmonds & Kiran, 2006), as L1 and L2 lexicons tend to overlap (Ansaldo & Saidi, 2014; Faroqi-Shah et al., 2010). In the study by Croft et al. (2010), transfer occurred in the opposite direction, meaning that therapy in the stronger language benefited the weaker language, without the authors being able to clearly explain the origin of this. This second theory is more restrictive for clinical practice, given that the patient's mother tongue may not be spoken, or even known, by the speech and language therapist (Croft et al., 2010).

To sum up, while a large number of studies and literature reviews have provided solid evidence that language dominance before the accident modulates TIL, there are fewer studies on the impact of language dominance after the accident. In all cases, taking language status into account highlights the importance of assessing pre-morbid skills using subjective questionnaires (*LEAP-Q - Language Experience and Proficiency Questionnaire*, Marian, Blumenfeld, & Kaushanskaya, 2007; *LHQ - Language History Questionnaire*, Li, Sepanski, & Zhao, 2006) and post-morbid abilities (Ansaldo & Saidi, 2014; Durand et al., 2018). Nickels, Hameau, Nair, Barr and Biedermann (2019) recall the importance of using assessment tools that are comparable across languages, such as the BAT.

1.2 Influence of the typological proximity of languages

Assuming that languages from the same family share linguistic representations because they are descended from the same parent language, it seems consistent that they allow greater cross-linguistic transfer (Kopke, 2013). Results in this direction

(Dieguez-Vide et al., 2012; Goral et al., 2007; Knoph, 2013; Knoph et al., 2015; Miertsch et al., 2009) support the general model of language production in bilinguals (De Bot, 2004) and confirm that other languages may be active to different degrees, simultaneously with the language chosen by the speaker at a given moment. Interference is assumed to be more frequent and more numerous between native languages because they are more likely to rely on similar processing (Kopke, 2013). According to Murphy (2003, cited in Dieguez-Vide et al., 2012), linguistic typology is one of the most important variables in the occurrence of TIL in bilinguals.

Contradictory results (Conner et al., 2018; Croft et al., 2010; Knoph, 2010; Marangolo et al., 2009) indicate that transfer is possible between very distant languages. In fact, linguistic similarities would put nearby languages in competition and make them less conducive to the appearance of TIL (Conner et al., 2018). The discussions are more contrasted in the literature reviews studied. In short, while Ansaldo and Saidi (2014) and Khachatryan et al. (2016) mention linguistic typology as a factor favouring TIL, Faroqi-Shah et al. (2010) reveal that it has very little differential effect on the results. Finally, Mosca (2017) advises the use of this variable with trilingual or polyglot individuals, with the aim of highlighting different patterns of linguistic recovery, depending on the typological proximity to the re-educated language. Recent clinical recommendations suggest that speech and language therapists assess the structural proximity of their patients' languages using specific didactic books; and possibly call on an interpreter if the languages are structurally distant (Durand et al., 2018).

1.3 Influence of the therapeutic approach

Theoretical models of language production predict that TIL is possible using semantic and phonological approaches (Croft et al., 2010). Nevertheless, the literature shows that the use of semantic therapy is more likely to lead to an improvement in the items treated (direct benefits), possible intra- and inter-linguistic generalisations (indirect benefits), and maintenance of acquisition over time (Faroqi-Shah et al., 2010). The hypothesis that semantic processing is more conducive to TIL than phonological processing has been fully or partially confirmed by Ansaldo and Saidi (2014), Croft et al. (2010) and Knoph et al. (2015). Since semantic aspects are thought to be common to the languages of a multilingual (Croft et al., 2010), the activation of a concept in a chosen language simultaneously extends to two separate lexicons in the two languages (Kiran & Iakupova, 2011) and thus activates semantically related words in these languages (Knoph et al., 2015). The impact of an intervention targeting the semantic system, such as SFA, is beneficial, despite inter-individual variability that sometimes makes it difficult to interpret the results (Kiran & Roberts, 2010). Initially developed for lexical retrieval, SFA has mostly been studied using nouns (Edmonds & Kiran, 2006; Kiran & Iakupova, 2011; Kiran & Roberts, 2010; Mung & Claivaz, 2016). Verb enhancement in unprocessed languages is therefore an important discovery today. If SFA processing of verbs favourably influences different linguistic levels, it would deserve to be reused in the future in other language contexts and could emerge as a promising treatment for PBaA (Knoph et al., 2015). According to the findings of Laganaro and Overton Venet (2001), TIL occurs only when processes common to the languages involved are targeted in therapy (i.e., when a task requires the same strategies in both languages). On the contrary, language benefits are limited to the language being treated when the treatment involves lexical or syntactic elements specific to that language.

Jaillet (2015) justifies this by the fact that bilinguals do not necessarily have the same lexicon in their two languages, because they use it differently in everyday life. Thus, re-educating a specific lexicon in one language will have little or no transfer effect if this same lexicon was not previously used or used very little in the other language. Clearly, targeting strategies shared by languages promote TIL (Lorenzen & Murray, 2008). Galvez and Hinckley (2003) and Conner et al. (2018) therefore recommend that future research use more general treatments such as SFA and ORLA.

1.4 Influence of the elements used in therapy

Three patterns of TIL are observed after the use of 'translation equivalents' (cognate words) in bilingual therapy: a facilitating effect of cognates, an inhibiting effect of cognates, or no effect (Hameau, 2013). Firstly, the advantage of cognates in PBaA, the most frequently found in studies, confirms the theoretical elements of Costa et al. (2005). The latter analysed and discussed Kohnert's (2004) study, explaining that the "cognate effect" in bilingual discourse production originates in the interdependence of the lexical and phonological levels. Firstly, when a word is produced, there would be phonological activation of the target word in the desired language, but also of its translation into the second language. The phonological content would therefore be activated from two sources. Secondly, the activation of phonological information would affect the lexical selection process, which in turn would activate all the words to which it is connected. Thus, the connections between lexical elements and phonological forms would be assumed to be bidirectional. These two processes are not ambivalent and interact within and between languages. Cognate words also cause a 'neighbourhood effect': during oral production, a target word activates words that are phonologically similar to it, i.e. differ by only one sound (Jaillet, 2015). Knowing that the processing of words with a dense linguistic neighbourhood is facilitated, the 'cognate effect' can obviously be seen as a special case of a 'neighbourhood effect' (Costa et al., 2005). At present, it remains difficult to distinguish whether the apparent effects are due to differences in the representation of words in the lexicon, or rather to a more general property of the speech production system. For Manolescu and Jarema (2018, p. 2), the differential action of cognate words compared to non-cognate words corroborates "the hypothesis of a functional link between the two languages of bilingual speakers."

Second, Kurland and Falcon (2011) reported an inhibitory effect of cognates with surprisingly higher overall performance for non-cognate words. In their patient, cognates acted as a distractor, rather than facilitating naming. As discussed in Abutalebi and Green's (2007) model of language selection and control, the choice of a target word necessarily involves lexical competition mediated by an inhibitory control mechanism. This patient's brain lesions were major, and according to Ansaldo and Saidi (2014), TIL potentiality for cognate words would tend to disappear if cognitive control circuits are damaged. In this case, the selection of the right word and the inhibition of competing words in other languages become impossible. A second explanation for this effect is that inhibition may be lifted in cerebral areas of the right hemisphere. However, it has been shown that the involvement, or even 'over-activation' of this hemisphere is not a good prognosis for aphasic recovery (Kurland & Falcon, 2011).

Third, from a more neutral perspective, Hameau and Kopke (2015) did not find any particular cognitive effect in TIL. Among several explanations based on theoretical work (Costa et al., 2005), the most convincing is that of a severe cerebral deficit at the sublexical level. "The connections between the two languages would have been "broken" phonologically, so that no "cognate effect" could be predicted in this patient". (Hameau, 2013, p. 94).

Despite some contradictory results, cognates justify the interest of exploiting multilingual lexico - semantic links in rehabilitation (Kohnert, 2004), with a view to maximising TIL (Lalor & Kirsner, 2001). Durand et al (2018) suggest that clinicians use the Dictionary of Cognates (Molina, 2011), which allows word lists to be drawn up that are similar between certain Latin languages. Further studies with other PBaAs should help elucidate the conditions under which this particular effect emerges (Hameau, 2013; Kurland & Falcon, 2011).

2   Limits

2.1 Limitations of the studies contained in the systematic review

The studies contained in the literature review proved to be very heterogeneous. Miller Amberber (2012) discusses, on the one hand, the differences in measures

On the one hand, there was a wide range of language assessment and treatment methods, and on the other, there was inter-individual diversity. In fact, the subjects in the case studies presented a variety of aphasiological deficits, as well as a type of bilingualism that was unique to them, in terms of age, history of acquisition and command of their languages. This singularity has often been presented as the main limitation of single cases (Ansaldo et al., 2010; Conner et al., 2018; Kiran & Iakupova, 2011; Kohnert, 2004; Marangolo et al., 2009; Radman et al., 2016) and multiple cases (Croft et al, 2010; Edmonds & Kiran, 2006); or despite a sometimes consequent sample (17 subjects), this did not reflect all possible combinations of ages of language acquisition, exposure and alteration/lesion (Kiran, Grasemann et al., 2013). In addition, a particular caveat should be placed on the impact of spontaneous recovery. A number of results could be biased by the presence of many aphasic subjects still in the acuteë phase of their cerebral accident (Costa et al., 2005; Faroqi- Shah et al., 2010; Kohnert, 2009). When certain experimental protocols begin less than six months after the onset of the accident, Kohnert (2009) explains that it is extremely difficult, if not impossible, to determine whether the generalisation of therapeutic benefits is a positive consequence of speech therapy or rather a reflection of spontaneous neurological recovery. For example, of the twelve studies included in the author's literature review, ten showed significant improvements in language in the untreated language. But in reality, six out of ten studies included subjects only a few weeks or months after cerebrolesion. This transitional phase may lead the patient to make spontaneous progress in his or her language(s), and may be mistakenly presented as a successful TIL. A final obstacle is the imprecision of certain studies concerning the patient's injury and language history.

2.2 Limitations of the systematic review

From a methodological point of view, there are several limitations. Firstly, the number of sources questioned remains limited. Additional databases should be explored to complete the research. The second limitation concerns the indexing of key words, as there is no consensus on what the main concept of the study should be called.

According to the list of key words in each study (Appendix C), the terms used are transfer, *therapy* transfer, *generalisation / generalization*, *treatment* generalisation, cross-language *transfer /* cross-linguistic transfer. The multitude of synonyms and the absence of specific MeSH terms may have distorted the results. The third bias was selection bias, as some articles could not be identified or retrieved from the databases. In addition, the lack of grey literature may expose our study to publication bias. Finally, overall, the selection, data extraction and article analysis processes were all carried out by a single reader, which may compromise fidelity.

3   Clinical perspectives for professional practice

The inventory of our results has made it possible to identify interesting perspectives for speech and language therapy practice. To date, the number of studies targeting the question of transfer of therapy between languages remains limited and research is probably still in its infancy. Given that a majority of the world's population is multilingual, and that this proportion is growing considerably, there is an urgent need for speech therapists to be better trained in the assessment and rehabilitation of bilingual aphasia (Faroqi-Shah et al., 2010) and to work in partnership with interpreters (Croft et al., 2010). Experimental data are needed in several languages to establish treatment protocols specific to bilingual aphasia (Miller Amberber, 2012) and to identify the particular conditions of cross-linguistic transfer in the case of monolingual therapy. In the meantime, Faroqi-Shah et al (2010) make the following recommendation: whenever the speech and language therapist has to make a decision about the choice of treatment, the L2 should be favoured - whatever the age of acquisition and the degree of competence - in accordance with the patient's linguistic preferences and the place of the language of the environment. This choice should not lead us to believe that treatment of L1 is detrimental to recovery, but rather that treatment of L2 in BPaA is currently considered to be effective (Faroqi-Shah et al., 2010; Kohnert, 2009; Laganaro, 2014). However, it is important to bear in mind that the generalisation of experience is more the exception than the norm (Nickels et al., 2019). In the near future, the joint analysis of aphasiological disorders, cognitive models of bilingualism and neuroimaging data will provide a better understanding of the mechanisms involved in cross-linguistic transfer, and above all the extent to which they interact (Ansaldo & Saidi, 2014).

V Conclusion

At a time when practitioners are faced with an increasing number of bilingual patients in France and throughout the world, the question of the generalisation of the effects of treatment from one language to the other in bilingual patients is of great importance in aphasiology. From a clinical point of view, understanding why treatment in one language does or does not improve the untreated language presents a real challenge for speech and language therapists, who always wish to restore the most global and functional communication in the shortest possible time. However, it is wise to remember that the bilingual's two languages are in constant interaction and that any neurological damage by definition makes bilingual aphasia unique (Khachatryan et al., 2016). The aim of this review of the literature was to identify the studies that have implemented monolingual rehabilitation in bilinguals with aphasia, and then to identify the various factors that influence the possible generalisation of learning from the re-educated language to the non-re-educated language.

A bibliometric search led to the selection, reading and analysis of twenty-six scientific articles. The heterogeneity of the results found in the literature shows that the question of rehabilitation of bilingual aphasia is complex and still divides researchers. A large number of studies show that, under certain conditions, a language can partially improve without first being reeducated. The status of the language being treated, the typological proximity of the languages, the nature of the therapy and the nature of the elements included in the therapeutic protocol are the main factors that can be influenced in the hope of encouraging this transfer. Other factors such as the place of the language of the environment, the role of an interpreter in the therapy, the intensity of the rehabilitation or the state of the cognitive control circuit also seem to modulate transfer to a lesser degree. In the current state of knowledge, these variables are beginning to be well identified and confirmed, but the way in which they interact with each other is still too poorly understood. In the coming years, speech and language therapists will need to be better prepared to deal with these multilingual patients.

Pending further publications on the subject, clinical recommendations have been proposed to help practitioners make the best therapeutic choice for their patients.

References

Abdelilah-Bauer, B. (2008). *Le défi des enfants bilingues: Grandir et vivre en parlant plusieurs langues* (La Decouverte). Paris, France.

Abutalebi, J., & Green, D. (2007). Bilingual language production: The neurocognition of language representation and control. *Journal of Neurolinguistics, 20*(3), 242-275. https://doi.org/10.1016/j.jneuroling.2006.10.003

Abutalebi, J., Rosa, P. A. D., Tettamanti, M., Green, D. W., & Cappa, S. F. (2009). Bilingual aphasia and language control: A follow-up fMRI and intrinsic connectivity study. *Brain and Language, 109*(2-3), 141-156. https://doi.org/10.1016/j.bandl.2009.03.003

Ansaldo, A. I., & Saidi, L. G. (2014). Aphasia therapy in the age of globalization: Cross- linguistic therapy effects in bilingual aphasia. *Behavioural Neurology, 2014*, 1-10. https://doi.org/10.1155/2014/603085

Ansaldo, A. I., Saidi, L. G., & Ruiz, A. (2010). Model-driven intervention in bilingual aphasia: Evidence from a case of pathological language mixing. *Aphasiology, 24*(2), 309-324. https://doi.org/10.1080/02687030902958423

Bardyn, N., & Martin, C. (2012). Predictive variables of recovery in 5 late bilingual aphasic patients. In P. Gatignol & S. Topouzkhanian, *Bilinguisme et biculture: Nouveaux défis?* (pp. 253-292). Isbergues, France: Ortho Edition.

Boyle, M., & Coehlo, C. A. (1995). Application of Semantic Feature Analysis as a Treatment for Aphasic Dysnomia. *American Journal of Speech-Language Pathology, 4*(4), 94-98. https://doi.org/1058-0360/95/0404-0094

Brin, F., Courrier, C., Lederle, E., Masy, V., & Kremer, J.-M. (2011). *Dictionnaire dorthophonie* (3rd edition). Paris, France: Ortho Edition.

Centeno, J. G., & Ansaldo, A. I. (2013). Aphasia in Multingual Populations. In I. Papathanasiou, P. Coppens, & C. Potagas, *Aphasia and Related Neurogenic Communication Disorders* (pp. 275-293). Burlington, Massachusetts: Jones & Bartlett Learning.

Cherney, L. R. (2004). Aphasia, alexia, and oral reading. *Topics in Stroke Rehabilitation, 11*(1), 22-36. https://doi.org/10.1310/VUPX-WDX7-J1EU-00TB

Chomel-Guillaume, S., Leloup, G., & Bernard, I. (2010). *Les aphasies: Evaluation et reeducation*. Issy-les-Moulineaux: Elsevier Masson.

Conner, P. S., Goral, M., Anema, I., Borodkin, K., Haendler, Y., Knoph, M., … Moeyaert, M. (2018a). The role of language proficiency and linguistic distance in cross-linguistic treatment effects in aphasia. *Clinical Linguistics & Phonetics, 32*(8), 739-757. https://doi.org/10.1080/02699206.2018.1435723

Costa, A., Santesteban, M., & Cano, A. (2005). On the facilitatory effects of cognate words in bilingual speech production. *Brain and Language, 94*(1), 94-103. https://doi.org/10.1016/j.bandl.2004.12.002

Costa, A., & Sebastian-Galles, N. (2014). How does the bilingual experience sculpt the brain? *NatureReviews . Neuroscience, 15*(5),336-345. https://doi.org/10.1038/nrn3709

Croft, S., Marshall, J., Pring, T., & Hardwick, M. (2010). Therapy for naming difficulties in bilingual aphasia: which language benefits? *International Journal of Language& Communication Disorders, 46*(1), 48-62.

https://doi.org/10.3109/13682822.2010.484845

Dana-Gordon, C., Mazaux, J.-M., & N'Kaoua, B. (2013). La prise en charge speech therapy for bilingual/multilingual aphasic patients: recent data. *Reeducation Orthophonique*, (253), 53-80.

Davis, G. A., & Wilcox, M. J. (1981). Incorporating parameters of natural conversation in aphasia treatment: PACE therapy. In R. Chapey (Ed.), *Language intervention strategies in adult aphasia* (pp. 169-193). Baltimore, MD: Williams & Wilkins.

De Bot, K. (2004). The Multilingual Lexicon: Modelling Selection and Control. *International Journal ofMultilingualism, 1*(1), 17-32. https://doi.org/10.1080/14790710408668176

Dieguez-Vide, F., Gich-Fulla, J., Puig-Alcantara, J., Sanchez-Benavides, G., & Pena-Casanova, J. (2012). Chinese-Spanish-Catalan trilingual aphasia: A case study. *JournalofNeurolinguistics, 25*(6),630-641. https://doi.org/10.1016/j.jneuroling.2012.01.002

Durand, E., Masson-Trottier, M., & Ansaldo, A. I. (2018). L'orthophoniste a l'ere de la globalisation : intervenir aupres des populations allophones souffrant d'aphasie. *Reeducation Orthophonique*, (275), 29-50.

Edmonds, L. A., & Kiran, S. (2006). Effect of Semantic Naming Treatment on Crosslinguistic Generalization in Bilingual Aphasia. *Journal of Speech, Language, and Hearing Research, 49*, 729-748.

EOLE (2003) familiesof famillesde langues. Reperea http://eole.irdp.ch/activites_eole/annexes_doc/annexe_doc_31.pdf

Fabbro, F. (2001). The Bilingual Brain: Bilingual Aphasia. *Brain and Language, 79*(2), 201-210. https://doi.org/10.1006/brln.2001.2480

Faroqi-Shah, Y., Frymark, T., Mullen, R., & Wang, B. Y. (2010). Effect of treatment for bilingual individuals with aphasia: A systematic review of the evidence. *Journal of Neurolinguistics, 23*(4),319-341. https://doi.org/10.1016/j.jneuroling.2010.01.002

Filiputti, D., Tavano, A., Vorano, L., De Luca, G., & Fabbro, F. (2002). Nonparellel recovery of languages in a quadrilingual aphasic patient. *International Journal of Bilingualism, 6*(4), 395-410. https://doi.org/10.1177/13670069020060040201

Galvez, A., & Hinckley, J. J. (2003). Transfer patterns of naming treatment in a case of bilingual aphasia. *Brain and Language, 87*(1),173-174. https://doi.org/10.1016/S0093-934X(03)00256-6

Gatignol, P., & Topouzkhanian, S. (Ed.). (2012). *Bilingualism and biculturalism: New challenges?* Isbergues, France: Ortho Edition.

Gil, M., & Goral, M. (2004). Nonparallel recovery in bilingual aphasia: Effects of language choice, language proficiency, and treatment. *International Journal of Bilingualism, 8*(2), 191-219. https://doi.org/10.1177/13670069040080020501

Gollan, T. H., Montoya, R. I., Fennema-Notestine, C., & Morris, S. K. (2005). Bilingualism affects picture naming but not picture classification. *Memory & Cognition, 33*(7), 1220-1234.

Goodglass, H., & Kaplan, E. (1972). *Assessment of Aphasia and Related Disorders*. Philadelphia, USA: Lea & Febiger.

Goral, M., Levy, E., & Kastl, R. (2007). Cross-language treatment generalization: A case of trilingual aphasia. *Brain and Language, 103*(1-2), 203-204. https://doi.org/10.1016/j.bandl.2007.07.116

Goral, M., Naghibolhosseini, M., & Conner, P. S. (2013). Asymmetric inhibitory treatment effects in multilingual aphasia. *Cognitive Neuropsychology, 30*(7-8), 564-577. https://doi.org/10.1080/02643294.2013.878692

Goral, M., Rosas, J., Conner, P. S., Maul, K. K., & Obler, L. K. (2012). Effects of language proficiency and language of the environment on aphasia therapy in a multilingual. *Journal ofNeurolinguistics, 25*(6), 538-551. https://doi.org/10.1016/j.jneuroling.2011.06.001

Grosjean, F. (2003). Le bilinguisme et le biculturalisme. Essai de definition. In A. Gorouben & B. Virole, *Le bilinguisme aujourd'hui et demain* (pp. 17-50). Paris, France: CTNERHI - GERS.

Grosjean, F. (2015). *Parler plusieurs langues: Le monde des bilingues.* Paris, France: Albin Michel.

Guilhem, V., Gomez, S., Prod'homme, K., & Kopke, B. (2013). Screening BAT: a rapid assessment tool available in 8 languages and adaptable to all BAT languages. *Reeducation Orthophonique,* (253), 121-142.

Guinel, N. (2013). De l'utilisation d'un dictaphone numerique en seances d'orthophonie pour des patients aphasiques bilingues. *Reeducation Orthophonique,* (253), 153-158.

Hameau, S. (2013). La prise en charge orthophonique du patient aphasique bilingue / multilingue: données recentes. *Reeducation Orthophonique,* (253), 81-97.

Hameau, S., & Kopke, B. (2015). Cross-language transfer for cognates in aphasia therapy with multilingual patients: a case study. *Aphasie und verwandte Gebiete | Aphasie et domaines associes, 2015*(3), 13-19.

Hughes, E., Roberts, J., & Tainturier, M. (2012). Cross-linguistic Generalisation of Treatment in Welsh-English Bilingual Anomia. *Procedia - Social and Behavioral Sciences, 61,* 168-169. https://doi.org/10.1016/j.sbspro.2012.10.131

Jaillet, C. (2015). *Code-switching: a means of facilitation for the bilingual aphasic? Case study of a bilingual Spanish-French aphasic patient* (Memoire d'Orthophonie, Universite Nice Sophia Antipolis). Reference https://dumas.ccsd.cnrs.fr/dumas-01497397/document

Khachatryan, E., Vanhoof, G., Beyens, H., Goeleven, A., Thijs, V., & Van Hulle, M. M. (2016). Language processing in bilingual aphasia: a new insight into the problem: Language processing in bilingual aphasia. *Wiley Interdisciplinary Reviews: Cognitive Science, 7*(3), 180-196. https://doi.org/10.1002/wcs.1384

Kiran, S., Grasemann, U., Sandberg, C., & Miikkulainen, R. (2013). A computational account of bilingual aphasia rehabilitation. *Bilingualism: Language and Cognition, 16*(2), 325-342. https://doi.org/10.1017/S1366728912000533

Kiran, S., & Iakupova, R. (2011). Understanding the relationship between language proficiency, language impairment and rehabilitation: Evidence from a case study. *Clinical Linguistics & Phonetics, 25*(6-7),565-583. https://doi.org/10.3109/02699206.2011.566664

Kiran, S., & Roberts, P. M. (2010). Semantic feature analysis treatment in Spanish-English and French-English bilingual aphasia. *Aphasiology, 24*(2), 231-261. https://doi.org/10.1080/02687030902958365

Kiran, S., Sandberg, C., Gray, T., Ascenso, E., & Kester, E. (2013). Rehabilitation in bilingual aphasia: Evidence for within- and between-language generalization. *American Journal of Speech-Language Pathology, 22*(2), S298-S309. https://doi.org/10.1044/1058-0360(2013/12-0085)

Knoph, M. (2010). Cross-Language Generalization in an Arabic-English Bilingual Person with Aphasia. *Procedia - Social and Behavioral Sciences, 6,* 208-209. https://doi.org/10.1016/j.sbspro.2010.08.104

Knoph, M. (2013). Intervention and Cross-language Transfer in Bilingual Aphasia - Two Single Case Studies. *Procedia - Social and Behavioral Sciences, 94,* 26-27. https://doi.org/10.1016/j.sbspro.2013.09.010

Knoph, M., Lind, M., & Simonsen, H. G. (2015). Semantic feature analysis targeting verbs in a quadrilingual speaker with aphasia. *Aphasiology, 29*(12), 1473-1496. https://doi.org/10.1080/02687038.2015.1049583

Kohnert, K. (2004). Cognitive and cognate-based treatments for bilingual aphasia: A casestudy . *BrainandLanguage, 91*(3),294-302. https://doi.org/10.1016/j.bandl.2004.04.001

Kohnert, K. (2009). Cross-language generalization following treatment in bilingual speakers with aphasia: A review. *Seminars in Speech and Language, 30*(03), 174-186. https://doi.org/10.1055/s-0029-1225954

Kopke, B. (2013). Bilingualism and aphasia. *Reeducation Orthophonique,* (253), 5-30.

Kopke, B., & Prod'homme, K. (2009). L'évaluation de l'aphasie chez le bilingue: une etude de cas. *Glossa, 107,* 39-50.

Kraetschmer, K. (1986). La reeducation de l'aphasique bilingue. *Communication Humaine Canada, 10*(3), 17-20.

Kroll, J. F., & Stewart, E. (1994). Category Interference in Translation and Picture Naming: Evidence for Asymmetric Connections between Bilingual Memory Representations. *Journal of Memory and Language, 33*(2),149-174. https://doi.org/10.1006/jmla.1994.1008

Kroll, Judith F., Dussias, P. E., Bice, K., & Perrotti, L. (2015). Bilingualism, Mind, and Brain. *AnnualReviewofLinguistics, 1*(1),377-394. https://doi.org/10.1146/annurev-linguist-030514-124937

Kung, J., Chiappelli, F., Cajulis, O. O., Avezova, R., Kossan, G., Chew, L., & Maida, C. A. (2010). From Systematic Reviews to Clinical Recommendations for Evidence-Based Health Care: Validation of Revised Assessment of Multiple Systematic Reviews (R-AMSTAR) for Grading of Clinical Relevance. *The Open Dentistry Journal, 4,* 84-91. https://doi.org/10.2174/1874210601004020084

Kurland, J., & Falcon, M. (2011). Effects of cognate status and language of therapy during intensive semantic naming treatment in a case of severe nonfluent bilingual aphasia. *Clinical Linguistics &Phonetics, 25*(6-7),584-600. https://doi.org/10.3109/02699206.2011.565398

Laganaro, M. (2014). Prise en charge de patients aphasiques bilingues dans leur deuxième langue, Second language treatment in bilingual aphasia. *Revue de neuropsychologie, me 6*(3), 207-210. https://doi.org/10.1684/nrp.2014.0310

Laganaro, M., & Overton Venet, M. (2001). Acquired Alexia in Multilingual Aphasia and Computer-Assisted Treatment in Both Languages: Issues of Generalisation and Transfer. *Folia Phoniatrica and Logopaedica, 53*(3),135-144.

https://doi.org/10.1159/000052668

Lalor, E., & Kirsner, K. (2001). The role of cognates in bilingual aphasia: Implications for assessment and treatment. *Aphasiology,* *15*(10-11),1047-1056. https://doi.org/10.1080/02687040143000384

Li, P., Sepanski, S., & Zhao, X. (2006). Language history questionnaire: A web-based interface for bilingual research. *Behavior Research Methods, 38*(2), 202-210.

Lorenzen, B., & Murray, L. L. (2008). Bilingual aphasia: A theoretical and clinical review. *American Journal of Speech-Language Pathology,* *17*(3), 299-317. https://doi.org/10.1044/1058-0360(2008/026)

Manolescu, A., & Jarema, G. (2018). Influence of grammatical gender and cognate status on the production of high-level bilinguals. *SHS Web of Conferences, 46*, 2-15. https://doi.org/10.1051/shsconf/20184610002

Marangolo, P., Rizzi, C., Peran, P., Piras, F., & Sabatini, U. (2009). Parallel recovery in a bilingual aphasic: a neurolinguistic and fMRI study. *Neuropsychology, 23(3)*, 405-409. https://doi.org/10.1037/a0014824

Marian, V., Blumenfeld, H. K., & Kaushanskaya, M. (2007). The Language Experience and Proficiency Questionnaire (LEAP-Q): Assessing language profiles in bilinguals and multilinguals. *Journal of Speech, Language, and Hearing Research, 50*(4), 940-967. https://doi.org/10.1044/1092-4388(2007/067)

Mazaux, J.-M., Pradat-Diehl, P., & Brun, V. (2007). *Aphasia and aphasics.* Issy-les-Moulineaux, France: Elsevier Masson.

Meinzer, M., Obleser, J., Flaisch, T., Eulitz, C., & Rockstroh, B. (2007). Recovery from aphasia as a function of language therapy in an early bilingual patient demonstrated by fMRI. *Neuropsychologia, 45*(6), 1247-1256. https://doi.org/10.1016/j.neuropsychologia.2006.10.003

Miertsch, B., Meisel, J. M., & Isel, F. (2009). Non-treated languages in aphasia therapy of polyglots benefit from improvement in the treated language. *Journal of Neurolinguistics,* *22*(2),135-150. https://doi.org/10.1016/j.jneuroling.2008.07.003

Miller Amberber, A. (2012). Language intervention in French-English bilingual aphasia: Evidence of limited therapy transfer. *Journal of Neurolinguistics, 25*(6), 588-614. https://doi.org/10.1016/j.jneuroling.2011.10.002

Moher, D., Liberati, A., Tetzlaff, J., Altman, D. G., & The PRISMA Group (2009). Preferred Reporting Items for Systematic Reviews and Meta-Analyses: The PRISMA Statement. *PLoSMedicine, 6*(7), e1000097. https://doi.org/10.1371/journal.pmed.1000097

Molina, R. M. (2011). *The Dictionary of Cognates* (1st edition). Cognates.org.

Mosca, M. (2017). *Multilinguals' Language Control.* Faculty of Human Sciences of the University of Potsdam, Potsdam, Germany.

Mung, S., & Claivaz, A. (2016). Comparison of anomia treatment in bilingual and monolingual therapy in an aphasic patient. *Aphasie und verwandte Gebiete | Aphasie et domaines associes, 42*(1), 27-40.

Nespoulous, J.-L., Joanette, Y., & Lecours, A.- R. (1986). *Protocole Montreal-Toulouse d'examen linguistique de l'aphasie (MT-86).* Isbergues, France: Ortho Edition.

Nickels, L., Hameau, S., Nair, V. K. K., Barr, P., & Biedermann, B. (2019). Ageing with bilingualism: benefits and challenges. *Speech, Language and Hearing, 22*(1), 32-50. https://doi.org/10.1080/2050571X.2018.1555988

Paradis, M. (1977). Bilingualism and Aphasia. In H. A. Whitaker & H. Whitaker (Ed.), *Studies in Neurolinguistics* (1st edition, Vol. 3, p. 65-121). New-York, EU: Academic Press.

Paradis, M. (1995). Bilingual aphasia - 100 years later: consensus and controversies. In M. Paradis (Ed.), *Aspects of bilingual Aphasia* (1st edition). Bingley, UK: Emerald Group Publishing Limited.

Paradis, M. (2000). Aphasia in bilinguals and multilinguals. In J.-A. Rondal & X. Seron, *Troubles du langage - Bases theoriques: diagnostics et reeducation* (new edition, p. 529 - 549). Liege, Belgium: Pierre Mardaga.

Paradis, M., & Libben, G. (1987). *The Assessment of Bilingual aphasia* (1st edition). Hillsdale, New Jearsey: Lawrence Earlbaum Associates.

Pulvermuller, F., Neininger, B., Elbert, T., Mohr, B., Rockstroh, B., Koebbel, P., & Taub, E. (2001). Constraint-induced therapy of chronic aphasia after stroke. *Stroke, 32*(7), 1621-1626.

Radman, N., Spierer, L., Laganaro, M., Annoni, J.-M., & Colombo, F. (2016). Language specificity of lexical-phonological therapy in bilingual aphasia: A clinical and electrophysiological study. *Neuropsychological Rehabilitation, 26*(4), 532-557. https://doi.org/10.1080/09602011.2015.1047383

Sabadell, V., Tcherniack, V., Michalon, S., Kristensen, N., & Renard, A. (2018). *Pathologies neurologiques: bilans et interventions orthophoniques* (1ere edition). Louvain-la-Neuve, Belgium: De Boeck Universite.

Santiago-Delefosse, M. (2004). Evaluating the quality of publications: What specificities for qualitative research? *Pratiques psychologiques, 10*(3), 243-254.

Schwieter, J., & Sunderman, G. (2009). Concept Selection and Developmental Effects in Bilingual Speech Production. *Language Learning, 59*, 897-927. https://doi.org/10.1111/j.1467-9922.2009.00529.x

Shea, B. J., Grimshaw, J. M., Wells, G. A., Boers, M., Andersson, N., Hamel, C., ... Bouter, L. M. (2007). Development of AMSTAR: a measurement tool to assess the methodological quality of systematic reviews. *BMC Medical Research Methodology, 7*, 10. https://doi.org/10.1186/1471-2288-7-10

Verreyt, N., De Letter, M., Hemelsoet, D., Santens, P., & Duyck, W. (2013). Cognate Effects and Executive Control in a Patient with Differential Bilingual Aphasia. *Applied Neuropsychology: Adult, 20*(3), 221-230. https://doi.org/10.1080/09084282.2012.753074

Zaugg, V., Savoldelli, V., Sabatier, B., & Durieux, P. (2014). Improving care practices and organisation: methodology of systematic reviews. *Sante Publique, 26*(5), 655-667.

APPENDICES

<u>APPENDIX A :</u>
*   Schematisation of the RHM model by Kroll and Stewart (1994)
*   Schematisation of the SbP model by Schwieter and Sunderman (2009)

<u>APPENDIX B:</u> General characteristics of the databases.

<u>APPENDIX C :</u>
*   Keywords used in the search.
*   Methods for querying sources and results.

<u>APPENDIX D:</u> Information table.

<u>APPENDIX E:</u> Examples of reading sheets.

<u>APPENDIX F :</u>
*   Presentation of the Santiago-Delefosse grid (2004)
*   Qualitative evaluation of single and multiple case studies (19 resources)

<u>APPENDIX G :</u>
*   Presentation of the AMSTAR grid by Shea et al (2007)
*   Qualitative assessment of literature reviews (7 resources)

<u>APPENDIX H:</u> Summary of the results of the literature search.

<u>APPENDIX I:</u> Studies that can be used in literature reviews.

<u>APPENDIX A:</u> Schematisation of theoretical models of language production.

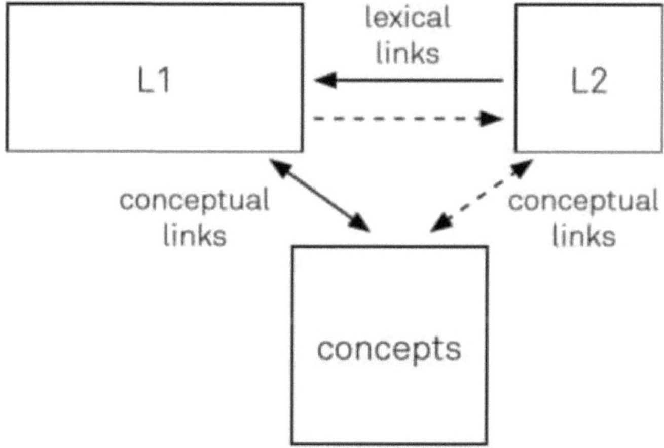

Figure 1: Modèle RHM (Kroll & Stewart, 1994)

"According to the RHM model (see Figure 1), the concepts of the bilingual subject are stored in an abstract semantic system common to both languages. On the other hand, the words of each language are stored in separate lexicons, following an organisation that presents several asymmetries. The lexicon of the first language (L1) is more developed than that of the second language (L2) and the lexical links are stronger from L2 to L1 than vice versa, which implies that the subject uses different access routes in his memory in order to find the appropriate lexicon in the desired language. Thus, when a bilingual translates a word from L2 to L1, he relies on lexical links, whereas when he translates a word from L1 to L2, he relies on conceptual mediation. Although many previous studies have supported the theory of this model, some research suggests the need to revise it following ambivalent results (described by Brysbaert and Duyck, 2009 and Kroll et al., 2010)". (Mung & Claivaz, 2016)

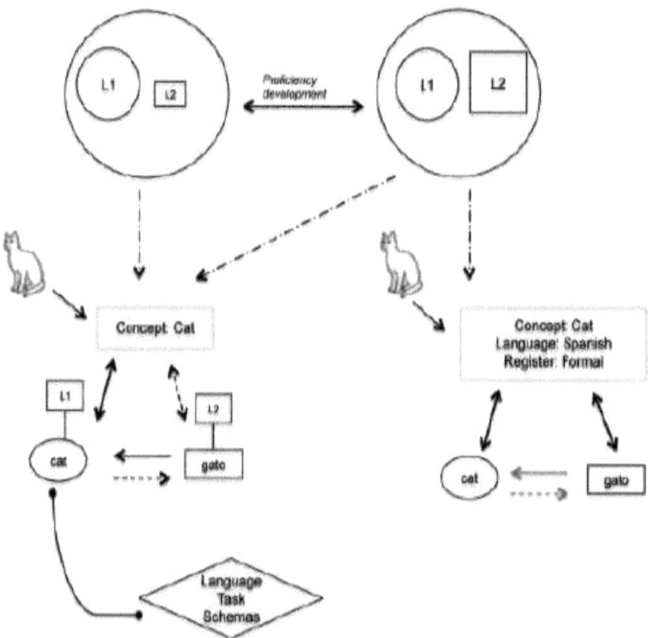

Figure 2: SbP model (Schwieter and Sunderman, 2009)

"A more recent model, the proficiency-based selection model (SbP, Schwieter and Sunderman, 2009) (see Figure 2) integrates the postulates of the RHM model and modulates them according to the speakers' proficiency level. It illustrates the active representations of a speaker naming an image in L2. The learners' level of proficiency is represented on a continuum from left (low proficiency) to right (high proficiency). For bilinguals with a low level of proficiency in their L2, there is a strong association between concepts and words in L1. On the other hand, the links between concepts and words in L2 are much weaker. As in the RHM model, learners are more dependent on lexical links than conceptual links when producing in L2.

Bilinguals must then go through the intermediary of the L1 lexicon in certain cases in order to produce a word in L2. In other words, the speaker will use lexical cues from the L1 to produce the word in L2. But in this case, a process of inhibition and activation also takes place. The intervention of control mechanisms is then required to inhibit competing words in the non-target language so that the appropriate word in the target language can be selected. In contrast, bilinguals with a high level of proficiency have a strong association between concepts and words in both L1 and L2. They are able to mediate conceptually in both languages, i.e. to use conceptual clues without having to use lexical clues from the other language to produce a word.

Moreover, they can rely on linguistic cues at the conceptual level that select the language of production (La Heij, 2005). Thus, the target word in the target language reaches the highest level of activation and is easily selected". (Mung & Claivaz, 2016)

APPENDIX B: General characteristics of the databases.

Database	Scope of intervention	Type of documents available
PubMed (English)	Biomedical and health sciences.	Periodical articles, book chapters.
ScienceDirect (English)	Technical, social, biomedical and health sciences.	Articles in periodicals, encyclopaedias, conference proceedings and summaries, book chapters, recommendations and guides to practice, etc.
Sudoc (French)	Higher education and research.	Books, journal articles, institutional work (theses, reviews).
LiSSa (French)	Public health.	Articles from periodicals.
ASHA (English)	Speech, language and hearing.	Periodical articles, recommendations and practice guides.

APPENDIX C :
- Keywords used for searches.

General concepts in French	English translation equivalents	Truncation may be used
Aphasia	Aphasia	Aphasi*
Bilingualism	Bilingualism Multilingualism Polyglot	Biling* Multingu* Polyglot* Bilingual* Multingu* Polyglot* Bilingual* Multingu* Polyglot
Reeducation	Rehabilitation Therapy / Therapies Intervention	
Inter-linguistic transfer	"Cross-linguistic transfer	
Child	Child / Children	

Methods for querying sources and results.

Database	How to search for sources	Details of search equations and filters used	Results obtained
PubMed (English)	Search equation based on MeSH terms. Filters.	(multilingu* OR bilingu* OR polyglot*) AND (aphasia OR "cross-linguistic transfer") AND (rehabilitation OR therapy OR	82 results [2000 - 2018] (19

		therapies OR intervention) NOT (child OR children) filters: 2000 to 2018 + Research articles	**retained)**
ScienceDirect (English)	Search equation based on MeSH terms. Filters.	"Aphasia; bilingualism; intervention filters: 2000 to 2018 + Research articles	85 results [2000 - 2018] **(5 deducted)**
Sudoc (French)	Advanced search. Thesaurus. Filters.	(multilingu* OR bilingu* OR polyglot*) AND (aphasia OR "cross-linguistic transfer") AND (rehabilitation OR therapy OR therapies OR intervention) NOT (child OR children)	3 results **(none withheld)**
LiSSa (French)	Simple search. Thesaurus.	Simple search: "aphasia and bilingualism".	4 results **(1 selected)**
ASHA (English)	Advanced search. Filters.	Search by domain > Speech-Language Pathologists > Practice Portal > Aphasia > Aphasia Evidence Map. filters : "Bilingual Considerations" > "Systematic Review	3 results **(2 retained)**

Date	Titre de l'article	Auteurs, Année	Source de parution de l'article	Secteur disciplinaire	Base de données et stratégies	Fiabilité de la BDD	Type d'étude et langue	Mots-clés de l'article
12.09.13	Prise en charge de patients aphasiques bilingues dans leur deuxième langue	Laganaro, 2014	"Revue de Neuropsychologie"	Neuropsychologie linguistique	Par mots-clés sur LiSSa. 1er résultat / 4.	Source reconnue Auteure référencée	Revue de littérature ; Français	aphasie bilingue, thérapie, L1, L2, transfert inter-langues
12.09.13	Cross-language transfer for cognates in aphasia therapy with multilingual patients: a case study	Hameau, Köpke, 2015	"Aphasie et Domaines Associés"	Aphasiologie	Part tre de l'article sur HAL ressource indiquée par un tiers.	Source reconnue Auteures référencées	Etude de cas unique ; Anglais	/
25.09.18	Effect of treatment for bilingual individuals with aphasia: A systematic review of the evidence	Faroqi-Shah, Frymark, Mullen, Wang, 2015	"Journal of Neurolinguistics"	Neurosciences Sciences du langage	Par arborescence sur ASHA. 2ème résultat / 3.	Source reconnue 3/4 auteurs référencés	Revue de littérature ; Anglais	aphasia bilingualist, cross-language transfer, multilingualism, speech-language pathologist
26.09.18	Parallel recovery in bilingual aphasia : A neurolinguistic and fMRI study	Marangolo, Rizzi, Peran, Piras, Sabatini, 2009	"Neuropsychology"	Neuropsychologie	Par écuation sur PubMed. 56ème résultat / 82.	Source reconnue 3/5 auteurs référencés	Etude de cas unique ; Anglais	bilingual aphasia, language recovery, language rehabilitation, naming, neuroimaging

37

Date	Titre de l'article	Auteurs, Année	Source de pertinence	Secteur disciplinaire	Base de données et st...	Fiabilité de la BDD	Type d'étude et langue	Mots-clés de l'article
25.09.18	**Rehabilitation in bilingual aphasia : Evidence for within- and between-language generalization**	**Kiran, Sandberg, Gray, Ascenso, Kester, 2013**	"American Journal of Speech-Language Pathology"	Médecine	Par équation sur PubMed 34ème résultat / 82.	Source reconnue Auteurs référencés	Etude de cas multiple ; Anglais	aphasia, bilingualism language disorders, neurologic disorders, intervention
01.10.18	**Aphasia therapy in the age of globalization : Cross linguistic therapy effects in bilingual aphasia**	**Ansaldo, Saidi, 2014**	"Behavioural Neurology"	Neurologie, Neuropsychologie, Neurosciences	Par équation sur PubMed 26ème résultat / 32. + Par dépouillement du DITO	Source reconnue :Auteurs référencés	Revue de littérature Anglais	aphasia, cross-language, generalization, cognates, naming treatment, transfer
06.10.18	**Cognitive and cognate-based treatments for bilingual aphasia : A case study**	**Kohnert, 2004**	"Brain and Language"	Neurologie, Neurosciences	Par équation sur PubMed 74ème résultat / 82. - Par mots-clés sur ScienceDirect. 74ème résultat / 85.	Source reconnue Auteure référencée	Etude de cas unique ; Anglais	bilingualism, language impairment, intervention, cross-linguistic cognates
11.10.18	**Comparaison du traitement de l'anomie dans une thérapie bilingue et monolingue chez une patiente aphasique**	**Mung, Claivaz, 2015**	"Aphasie : Domaines Associés"	Aphasiologie	Par titre de l'article sur ResearchGate : ressource indiquée par un des auteurs référencées	Source reconnue 1 / 2 auteurs référencées	Etude de cas unique ; Français	aphasie bilingue, traitement de l'anomie, généralisation intralangue et interlangue thérapie par analyse des traits sémantiques

Date	Titre de l'article	Auteurs, Année	Source de parution	Secteur disciplinaire	Base de données et …	Fiabilité de la EDD	Type d'étude et langue	Mots-clés de l'article
16.10.18	On the facilitatory effects of cognate words in bilingual speech production	Costa, Santesteban, Caño, 2005	"Brain and Language"	Neurobiologie, Neurosciences	Par titre de l'article sur ScienceDirect : dépouillement de bibliographie d'article.	Source reconnue Auteurs référencés	Discussion sur une étude de cas unique (Kohnert, 2004) ; Anglais	bilingualism, cognates, speech production aphasia
26.10.18	Semantic feature analysis targeting verbs in a quadrilingual speaker with aphasia	Knoph, Lind, Simonsen, 2015	"Aphasiology"	Aphasiologie	Par titre de l'article sur ResearchGate : dépouillement de bibliographie d'article.	Source reconnue Auteures référencées	Etude de cas unique ; Anglais	aphasia, multilingua, cross-linguistic transfer, semantic feature analysis (SFA), verb, action naming
20.11.18	Model-driven intervention in bilingual aphasia : Evidence from a case of pathological language mixing	Ansaldo, Saidi, Ruiz, 2010	"Aphasiology"	Aphasiologie	Par titre de l'article sur Taylor and Francis Online : dépouillement de bibliographie d'article.	Source reconnue Auteures référencées	Etude de cas multiple ; Anglais	bilingua aphasia, intervention, mode-based, pathological switching
27.11.18	Cross-language treatment generalisation : A case of trilingual aphasia.	Goral, Levy, Kastl, 2007	"Brain and Language"	Neurologie, Neurosciences	Par équation sur PubMed. 65ème résulta : /82.	Source reconnue Auteures référencées	Etude de cas unique ; Anglais	/
29.11.18	Cross-language generalization following treatment in bilingual speakers with aphasia : A review.	Kohnert, 2009	"Seminars in Speech and Language"	Sciences du langage	Par équation sur PubMed. 53ème résulta : /82. + Par arborescence sur ASHA. 3ème résulta : /3	Source reconnue Auteure référencée	Revue de littérature ; Anglais	aphasia bilingual, cross-linguistic transfer, intervention

Dat	Titre de l'article	Auteurs, Anné	Source de parution	Secteur disciplinaire	Base de données et	Fiabilité de la BDD	Type d'étude et langu	Mots-clés de l'article
15	06.12.18	Recovery from aphasia as a function of language therapy in an early bilingual patient demonstrated by fMRI.	Meinzer, Obleser, Flaisch, Eulitz, Rockstroh, 2007	"Neuropsychologia"	Neuropsychologie, Neurosciences	Par équation sur PubMed. 67ème résultat / 82.	Source reconnue Auteurs référencés	Etude de cas unique ; Anglais	language disorder, stroke, bilingualism, treatment, functional imaging
16	20.12.18	Effects of language proficiency and language of theenvironment on aphasia therapy in a multilingual.	Goral, Rosas, Conner, Maul, Obler, 2012	"Journal of Neurolinguistics"	Neurosciences, Sciences du langage	Par équation sur PubMed. 38ème résultat / 82. • Par mots-clé sur Science Direct. 38ème résultat / 85.	Source reconnue Auteurs référencés	Etude de cas unique ; Anglais	aphasia, BAT, cross-language, generalization, multilingual, treatment
17	20.12.18	Bilingual Aphasia : A theoretical and clinical review.	Lorenzen, Murag, 2008	"American Journal of Speech-Language Pathology"	Orthophonie	Par équation sur PubMed. 59ème résultat / 82. • Ressource indiquée par un tiers.	Source reconnue Auteures référencées	Revue de littérature ; Anglais	aphasia, bilingual, recovery, assessment, treatment
18	03.12.18	Language specificity of lexical-phonological therapy in bilingual aphasia : A clinical and electrophysiological study.	Radman, Spierer, Laganaro, Annoni, Colombo, 2016	"Neuropsychological Rehabilitation"	Neuropsychologie	Par équation sur PubMed. 22ème résultat / 82.	Source reconnue Auteures référencées	Etude de cas unique ; Anglais	bilingual aphasia, lexical-phonological therapy, cross language generalisation, brain lesion
19	03.12.18	Effects of cognate status and language of therapy during intensive semantic naming treatment in a case of severe nonfluent bilingual aphasia.	Kurland, Falcon, 2011	"Clinical Linguistics & Phonetics"	Linguistique, Orthophonie	Par équation sur PubMed. 45ème résultat / 82.	Source reconnue Auteures référencées	Etude de cas unique ; Anglais	bilingualism, aphasia, cognates, cross-linguistic generalization, intensive language therapy, constraint-induced language therapy

	Date	Titre de l'article	Auteurs, Ann	Source de parution	Secteur disciplinaire	Base de données et	Fiabilité de la BDD	Type d'étude et lang.	Mots-clés de l'article
20	03.12.18	Understanding the relationship between language proficiency, language impairment and rehabilitation : Evidence from a case study	Kiran, Iakupova, 2011	"Clinical Linguistics & Phonetics"	Linguistique, Orthophonie	Par équation sur PubMed. 46ème résultat / 82.	Source reconnue Auteures référencées	Etude de cas multiple ; Anglais	aphasia, bilingualism, assessment, treatment
21	14.01.19	Therapy for naming difficulties in bilingual aphasia: which language benefits ?	Croft, Marshall, Pring, Hardwick, 2010	"International Journal of Language and Communication Disorders"	Linguistique, Orthophonie	Par équation sur PubMed. 50ème résultat / 82.	Source reconnue Auteurs référencés	Etude de cas multiple ; Anglais	aphasia, bilingualism, case series, speech-and-language therapy
22	14.01.19	The role of language proficiency and linguistic distance in cross-linguistic treatment effects in aphasia.	Conner, Goral, Anema, Borodkin, Haendler, Knoph, Mustelier, Paluska, Melnikova, Moegaert, 2018	"Clinical Linguistics & Phonetics"	Linguistique, Orthophonie	Par équation sur PubMed. 1er résultat / 82.	Source reconnue Auteurs référencés	Etude de cas unique ; Anglais	multilingual, aphasia, cross-linguistic, language mixing, treatment generalisation, efficiency
23	14.01.19	Language processing in bilingual aphasia : a new insight into the problem.	Khachatryan, Vanhoof, Beyens, Goeleven, Thijs, Van Hulle, 2016	"Wiley Interdisciplinary Reviews: Cognitive Science'	Sciences cognitives	Par équation sur PubMed. 14ème résultat / 82.	Source reconnue Auteurs référencés	Revue de littérature ; Anglais	/

Date	Titre de l'article	Auteurs, Année	Source de parution	Secteur disciplinaire	Base de données et résultat	Fiabilité de la BDD	Type d'étude et langue	Mots-clés de l'article
15.01.19	A computational account of bilingual aphasia rehabilitation.	Kiran, Grasemann, Sandberg, Miikkulainen, 2013	"Bilingualism : Language and Cognition"	Linguistique, Multilinguisme, Neurosciences	Par équation sur PubMed. 30ème résultat / 82.	Source reconnue Auteurs référencés	Etude de cas multiple ; Anglais	computational modeling, rehabilitation, bilingual aphasia, generalization
15.01.19	Acquired alexia in multilingual aphasia and computer-assisted treatment in both languages : Issues of generalisation and transfer.	Laganaro, Overton Venet, 2001	"Folia Phoniatrica et Logopaedica"	Phoniatrie, Orthophonie	Par équation sur PubMed. 81ème résultat / 82.	Source reconnue Auteures référencées	Etude de cas unique ; Anglais	alexia, aphasia, treatment, bilingual, computerized
13.02.19	Language intervention in French-English bilingual aphasia : Evidence of limited therapy transfer	Miller Amberber, 2012	"Journal of Neurolinguistics"	Neurosciences, Sciences du langage	Par mots-clés sur ScienceDirect. 42ème résultat / 85.	Source reconnue Auteure référencée	Revue de littérature + étude de cas unique ; Anglais	bilingual aphasia, BAT generalisation, treatment cross-linguistic assessment, therapy transfer
25.02.19	Intervention and cross-language transfer in bilingual aphasia - Two single case studies.	Knoph, 2013	"Procedia - Social and Behavioral Sciences"	Psychologie, Sciences sociales	Par mots-clés sur ScienceDirect. 31ème résultat / 85.	Source reconnue Auteure référencée	Etude de cas multiple ; Anglais	/

- Presentation of the Santiago-Delefosse grid (2004)

STUDY		INTERVENTION		RESULTS		
Author Year, Source	Title of the study, Objectives	Population studied	Protecole ^intervention: type of study and speech therapy treatment	Immediate	Generalisation	Conclusion and limitations
Laganaro. 2014. Review of literature. -> 10 studies published between 2001 and 2014 (Revue de Neuropsychologic)	Management of **patients with aphasia who are bilingual in their** second **language.** Objective: To show: -If there is evidence on the eflkadte of the management of the fable language in bilingual patients -If the reeducation of the L2 has aussl effects on the L1.	11 bilingual adult patients. Age/sex/level of education: no information in the M-A but specified in each item individually. Variable language families: Romanic, Slavic Germanic, Indo-Iranian. Aphasias: no indication of the type and severity found in the M-A but specified in each article individually.	Reeducation unilingue diverse reeducation of Г anomie, alexia rehabilitation, lexico-phonological therapy. semantic therapy (SFA) constraint therapy (GIAT), etc. Rehabilitation frequency: no indicalions.	-Improvement of the processed language (L2) for the studies analysed.	-Generalisation (TIL) parlielle ou lotale a la langue non-lraitee (L1) pour 5 etudes /10. -No generalisation to L1 for 5/10 studies, or even pejoration of L1 or L2 for 2/10 studies.	Results - Effective **therapy** in L2. **-Transfer of** profits **L2 ->L1 not insured and seems to be** l i mite have **special** conditions such as: . **structural similarities between** languages (e.g. with **ph analogically similar** words or **cognate words) . when the therapy targets processes or representations shared by L2** and **L1.** Limits : -Studies requiring validation on a larger scale (number of cases studied limits -Variability in bilingual situations.
2015. Unique case study. (Aphasia and associated Dorna nes)	Cross-language transfer **for** cognates in aphasia therapy with multilingual patients: **a** case study. Objective: To examine the transfer of the benefits of therapy from one argument to another, with the hypothesis of a post-lexical criticism of the Гeffet cognat.	Man aged 71, right-hand man. very insiruii Triingue German (LI), English (L2) and French (L3). Very good pre-mcrbid ora as and ecrtes skills in these 3 languages. Non-fluent aphasia severe lesion following ischemic sy vie nr e gauctie. "roubles langsgiers: comprehension preserved. but sporrtanee expression ires redurte, with stereotypy and nec ogisms Efficacrte de 1 irdicagE phcnclcgique dans la denom nation. Reoetticn hindered by nee ogisms Speech therapy carried out in French, 4 times a week.	Study carried out at **28** words post-lesion 3 phases: 1} Evaluation laraeg ЕГЕ pre-irsitement In LI (German) and L3 (French): "■avec e BAT "avec иra tactie de denom "Out of 50 words . "5 words cognats franais-arg ais-a lemanc . "5 French cognates - al emend . 2C Nor-Cognais words "Out of 35 non-ertrafnes words (= words in the middle) 2)" 'base de tratemert PEC intensive en L3 (francais) -> therapie lex CD-SEP˙ anticue base sur 50 mots cognats. 27 sessions of 45min to 1h each, 1 or 2 fbis per icjr, 5 DLrS"7 for 3 weeks. 3} Evaluation largag ere post-trartemerrt : In LI (German) and L3 (French): "avec e BAT "avec ure tactie	-Amelioration of all French words (L3) : 25 -Legere amel oration des mots ■rancais ncn- ertra)nes (= mots oortrclesj: 12%	-Generalisation (TIL) for equivalents er al emend of words processed in French (cognates): 16%. The effects are more pronounced for words that come out of the cognates in the three languages. -Generalisation (TIL) of non-ocgrBts ei ron-ertrafnes German words: 14	Resullats : ■Benefits for words processed in L3 And **to a lesser** degree for words **not** processed **in** LI st L3. - **No** effect of cognates observed. -The results **seem** compatible **with** models **of** bilingual IExicalE production involving a strong interactivity of the different levels of intra- **and inter-language** representation **and** postulating a post-lexical origin of Г-effet cognat. -Proven effectiveness **of** naming **treatment** in **bilingual** aphasia **(particularly in the** chronic stage) **and** the potential for **TIL** in the

			de denom		untreated language. Li mites -ifncile ce liter des conclusions quant au statul CES langues traitees et non traitees car difficile de cire que les etaient LES langues les plus fortes et tai Dies du patient.

<u>APPENDIX F :</u>

- Presentation of the Santiago-Delefosse grid (2004)

Criteria to be assessed	*Operationalisation in qualitative research*
The research question	Q1 - Is it clearly defined? Q2 - If the question comes from the field and the empirical material, is it explicit at the end of the research process?
The search procedure	**-The research context** Q3 - Is it sufficiently described to enable the reader to follow and transpose the results to other similar settings? - **Methodology** Q4 - Is it appropriate to the question posed? Are other possible methods being considered/discussed? Q5 -Is each stage of the research described and illustrated (if necessary)? Q6 - Putting theoretical references into perspective? - **Sampling** Q7 -Is its constitution described and justified? Q8 - Does it include different possible cases in order to allow generalisations in similar settings? Q9 -Does it include a search for cases that contradict the analysis or modify the analysis if the sample is extended?
The theoretical reference framework	Q10 -Is it described in a way that is relevant to the research, and put into perspective with other work? Discussed and linked to the methodology?
Analysis and results (1/2)	Q11 - Is it clearly described and theorically justified? Is it related to the research question (and not an abusive generalisation given the empirical material)? Q12 - Does it present the links and articulations between empirical data and theoretical explanations in a coherent way?
Criteria to be evaluated	*Operationalisation in qualitative research*
Analysis and results (2/2)	Q13 - Can the results be reviewed by other peers (a-t-　　waves)?　　data　　empirical data or　　available, transcriptions, etc.)? Q14 - Does it take all the comments into account? Q15 - Does it explain the negative cases that may contradict or modify the results? Are they discussed with relevance and honesty?
Validity, Fidelity, Reflexivity of research work	Q16 - Is the analysis est-elle　　repeatedby　severalresearchers independent? Q17 - Did the research plan to obtain data through different channels, so that the data from the field could be cross-referenced? Q18 - Did the analysis make use of statistical verification (if appropriate to the research question, and if the material is suitable)? Computer processing? Q19 - Do we have enough details of the way we work, the empirical data and the validation research to convince a sceptical reader of the relationship between interpretations and results? Q20 - Is there any discussion of possible biases and the impact of the

	methods used on the data obtained? Is there any discussion of the ethical aspects of the research and their impact? Q21 - Are researchers capable of abstracting themselves from their research preconceptions?
Aim of the research	Q22 - Does research contribute to the production of useful knowledge for the discipline?

Qualitative evaluation of single and multiple case studies (19 resources).

Author of 1 study (year)	01M	Q171	Q171	Q4V1	QE[V1	QtfVI	QTVI	QtfVI	QfVI	Q10M	Q11M	Q12M	Q13M	Q14M	Q1ET7I	Q16M	Q17 J	Q18M	Q13M	Q20M	□21	'52'	Total	[VI]
Harneau, Kopke (2015)	0	0	0	0	0	0	0	N	N	0	0	0	0	0	0	N	0	0	0	0	0	0	19	86%
Marangolo, Rizzi, Peran, Piras, Sabatini (2009)	0	0	0	0	N	0	0	N	0	0	0	0	0	N	0	N	N	0	0	0	0	0	17	
Kiran, Sandberg, Gray, Ascenso, Kester (2013)	0	0	0	0	0	0	0	0	N	0	0	0	0	0	0	N	N	0	0	0	0	0	19	86%
Koh nert (2004)	0	0	0	0	0	0	0	N	N	0	0	0	0	0	0	N	0	0	0	0	0	0	19	66%
Mung, Claivaz (2016)	0	0	0	0	0	0	0	N	N	0	0	0	0	0	0	N	0	0	0	0	0	0	19	66%
Knoph, Lind, Simonsen (2015)	0	0	0	0	0	0	0	N	N	0	0	0	0	0	0	0	N	0	0	0	0	0	19	66%
Ansaldo, Saidi, Ruiz (2010)	0	0	0	0	0	N	0	0	0	0	0	0	0	0	0	0	N	0	0	0	0	0	20	91%
Goral, Levy, Kastl (2007)	0	0	0	0	N	N	0	N	N	N	0	N	N	N	N	N	N	0	N	N	0	0	9	41%
Meinzer, Obleser, Flaisch, Eulitz, Rockstroh (2007)	0	0	0	0	0	0	0	N	N	0	0	0	0	0	N	N	N	0	0	0	0	0	17	77%
Goral, Rosas, Conner, Maul, 0 bier (2012)	0	0	0	0	0	0	0	N	0	0	0	0	0	0	0	0	N	0	0	0	0	0	20	91%
Radman, Spierer, Laganaro, Annoni, Colombo (2016)	0	0	0	0	0	0	0	N	0	0	0	0	0	0	0	0	0	0	0	0	0	0	21	95%
Kurland, Falcon (2011)	0	0	0	0	0	0	0	N	N	0	0	N	0	0	0	N	N	0	0	0	0	0	17	77%
Kiran, Iakupova (2011)	0	0	0	0	N	0	0	N	0	0	0	0	0	N	0	N	N	0	0	0	0	N	16	73%
Croft, Marshall, Pring, Hardwick (2010)	0	0	0	0	0	0	0	0	0	0	0	0	0	0	0	0	0	0	0	0	0	0	22	100%
Conner, Goral, An ema, Borodkin, Haendler, Knoph, Mustelier, Paluska, Melnikova, Moeyaert (201S)	0	0	0	0	0	0	0	N	0	0	0	0	0	0	0	0	0	0	0	0	0	0	21	95%
Kiran, Grasemann, Sandberg, Miikkulainen (2013)	N	0	0	0	0	0	0	0	0	0	0	0	0	N	0	N	0	0	0	0	0	0	19	86%
Laganaro, Overton Venet (2001)	0	0	0	0	0	0	0	N	N	N	0	N	0	0	N	N	0	0	0	0	0	0	16	73%
Miller Amberber (2012)	0	0	0	0	0	N	0	N	N	0	0	0	0	0	N	0	N	0	0	0	0	0	17	77%
Knoph (2013)	0	0	N	0	N	0	0	N	N	0	N	N	N	N	N	N	N	N	N	N	N	0	7	32%
Average number of items =																							80%

APPENDIX G :

- Presentation of the revised R-AMSTAR grid (Kung et al., 2010), based on the initial AMSTAR grid (Shea et al., 2007).

1. Is an a priori research plan provided?

The research question and the inclusion criteria for the studies must be determined before the start of the review.

Criteria	Score:
A. Publication and/or registration of the study protocol in advance B. Description of inclusion criteria C. Well-targeted research question (PICO criteria) *Conditions for awarding the score* 3 criteria->4, 2-"3, I-"2,0->1 *Explanation A.:* It must be explicitly stated that the protocols have ёгё рнвпё or registered, for example in PROSPERO, a prospective and multinational online register of systёmatic journals. C. The question contains the PICO criteria, i.e. Population, Intervention (or exposure), Comparator (or controls) and Results *(Outcomes).*	Commentary:

2. Were at least two people responsible for selecting the studies and extracting the data?

At least two people must extract the data independently, and a consensus method must be in place to settle disputes.

Criteria	Score:
A. Data extracted by at least two people, independently ^ explicit or implicit declaration) B. Statement on the consensus process for settling disputes C. Resolution of disagreements between persons having extracted data in accordance with the established	Commentary:

method (explicit or implicit declaration)
Conditions for awarding the score
3 criteria-"4,2-"3, I-"2,0->I

---

3. Was the documentary research exhaustive?

At least two electronic sources must have been used. The report should include the time frame of the search and the databases searched (e.g. Central, EM BASE and MEDLINE). All searches should be completed by consulting the tables of contents of recent scientific journals, reviews of the literature, textbooks, specialised registers or experts in the field under study and by examining the references provided in the listed studies.

CriteriaScore :

A.   At least two electronic sources have been identified.   Comm entair e :
used.

B.   The time horizon and databases queried are indicated.

C.   Key words and/or MeSH terms are indicated and, where possible, the search strategy is outlined.

D. All research is completed by consulting the tables of contents of recent scientific journals, literary reviews, textbooks and registers, and by examining the references provided in the studies listed.

E. A manual search has been carried out in
magazines.

Scoring conditions
4 or 5 triteres-*4, 3-e3,2-*2,1 or D--!

Explanation E. :
The manual search consists of identifying the most relevant journals and manually searching their content, page by page, to identify any eligible studies.

---

4. Was the nature of the publication (grey literature, for example) a criterion for inclusion?

Authors should indicate whether they have searched for all reports, regardless of publication type, or whether they have excluded any reports (from their systematic review) on the basis of publication type, language, etc.

Criteria	Score:
A. The authors indicate that they have researched all the reports, regardless of the type of publication.	Commentary:
B. Authors indicate whether they have excluded reports on the basis of type of publication, language, etc.	
C. "Articles written in a language other than Γ English have been translated" or readers misunderstood the language of the report quite well.	
D. No restrictions based on language or consideration of articles written in a language other than English	
Conditions for awarding the score	
3 or 4 criteria-4, 2-"3, 1-2,0-1	

---

5. Is a list of studies (included and excluded) provided?

A list of included and excluded studies must be provided.

Criteria   Score:

A.   The studies included must be brought together in a Commentary: a table, a list or a figure; a simple list of references is not sufficient.

B.   Excluded studies must be compiled in a table, list or figure to be included in the article or supplement.

C.   The reasons for excluding studies that have been seriously considered must be explained clearly enough.

D.   The reader can easily trace the studies included and excluded in the bibliography, references or supplement to the article.

Conditions for awarding the score
4 criteria-*4, 3-3, 2-"2,1-*1

Here's how it works:

Excluded studies are those which, after having been seriously considered on the basis of the title and/or abstract, have been re-evaluated after reading the body of the text.

---

6. Are the characteristics of the studies included indicated?

Data on the subjects who took part in the original studies, the interventions they received and the results should be grouped together, for example in tabular form. Data on the characteristics of subjects in all the studies analysed (e.g. age, race, sex, relevant socio-economic data, nature, duration and severity of disease, other diseases) should y included.

Criteria	Score:
A. Data on the subjects who took part in the original studies, the interventions they responded to and the results are grouped together, in table form, for example.	Commentary:

B.   The authors describe the extent of the data on the relevant characteristics of the subjects in the studies analysed.

C.   The information provided seems complete and accurate.

Conditions for awarding the score

3 criteria->4, 2->3, I-"2,0->I

---

7.   Has the scientific quality of the <u>studies included </u>been assessed and recorded?

The evaluation methods determined a priori must be indicated (for example, for studies of practical effectiveness, the choice to include only randomised double-blind placebo-controlled clinical trials or to include only studies in which the allocation of subjects to study groups was concealed); for other types of study, other evaluation criteria will have to be taken into consideration.

CriteriaScore:

A.   A priori methods are indicated.   Commentary:

B.   The scientific quality of the studies included seems valid.

C.   The level of evidence is exposed, duly recognised or taken into consideration.

D.   The quality of the evidence is assessed or graded based on evidence evaluation tools.

Conditions for awarding the score

4 criteria-"4, 3->3, 2-"2,1 or O->1

Explanations D.:

An evidence assessment tool is an instrument used to establish the level of evidence. E.g. GRADE *(Grading of Recommendations Assessment, Development and Evaluation).*

---

8.   Has the scientific quality of the studies included in the review been used appropriately in formulating the conclusions?

The results of the evaluation of the methodological rigour and scientific quality of the included studies must be taken into account in the analysis and conclusions of the review, and explicitly formulated in the recommendations.

Criteria	Score :
A. The authors have taken scientific quality into account in the analysis and conclusions of the review.	Commentary:
B. Scientific quality is explicitly stated in the recommendations.	
C. The conclusions are geared towards the production of practice guides.	
D. Ґёnoncё clinical consensus suggests revision or confirmation of practice recommendations.	

Conditions for awarding the score

4 criteria-"4, 3->3, 2-"2,1 or O->1

---

9.   Are the methods used to combine the results of the studies appropriate?

If the results of the studies are to be combined, a homogeneity test must be carried out to ensure that they can be combined (chi-square or I^2 , for example). If there is heterogeneity, a random effects model must be used and/or it must be checked whether the nature of the clinical data justifies the combination (is the combination reasonable?).

CriteriaScore:

A.   The authors set out the criteria on the basis of which they determined that the studies analysed were similar enough to be combined.

B.   In the case of pooled results, the authors performed a homogeneity test to ensure that the studies could be combined.

C.   The authors have taken note of the heterogeneous nature (or otherwise) of the studies.

D.   If there was heterogeneity, the authors used a random effects model and/or checked whether the nature of the data justified the combination.

E.   If there is homogeneity, the authors explain the justification or the statistical test.

Conditions for awarding the score

4 or 5 criteria-"4,3-*3,2-"2,1 or 0-"I

---

10.   Has the likelihood of publication bias been assessed?

An assessment of publication bias should include a combination of graphical tools (study scatter diagram or other test) and/or statistical tests (Egger regression test, for example).

Criteria	Score:
A. Taking account of publication bias or the drawer effect	Comme
B. Graphical tools (e.g. study scatter diagrams)	

C.   Statistical tests (Egger regression test, for example)

Conditions for awarding the score

3 criteria-M, 2-"3,1->2,0->1

11.   Have any conflicts of interest been declared?

Possible sources of support must **be** declared, both for the systematic review and for the studies included.

Criteria	Score:
A. Presentation of sources of support	Commentary:
B. Absence of conflict of interest - We are dealing here **with** subjectivity; we may need to y alien by deduction or dig a little deeper.	
C. Inclusion or disclosure of sources of support or conflicts of interest in the **main** studies included	
Conditions for awarding the score	
3 criteria->4,2->3, I-"2,0->I	

- Qualitative assessment of literature reviews (7 resources).

Author of study (year)	Q1	Q2 v	Q3 -	Q4 '	Q5 v	Q6 '	Q7 '	QB '	Q9 - Q10 - Q11 v	Total/44 Я % '
Lorenzen, Muray (2008)	1	2	1	1	1	1	1	3	111	14	32%
Kohnert (2009)	3	Г1	3 2		1	4	1	1	111	19	43%
Faroqi-Shah, Frymark. Mullen. Wang (2010)	3	4	4	3 2		4	3	3	313	33	75%
Miller Amberber (2011)	1	1	1	1	1	4	1	2	312	18	41%
Ansaldo. Saidi (2014)	3	2	3 2		1	4	3	1	11 2	23	52%
Laganaro (2014)	2	Г1	1	1	1	3	1	2	112	16	36%
Khachatryan, Vanhoof, Beyens. Goeleven. Thijs, Van Hulle (2016)	3	2	1	2	1	2	1	1	11 2	17	39%
Average number of items =										I⁴⁵ % .

<u>**APPENDIX H:**</u> **Summary of the results of the literature search.**
Flow chart - PRISMA 2009 (Moher et al., 2009)

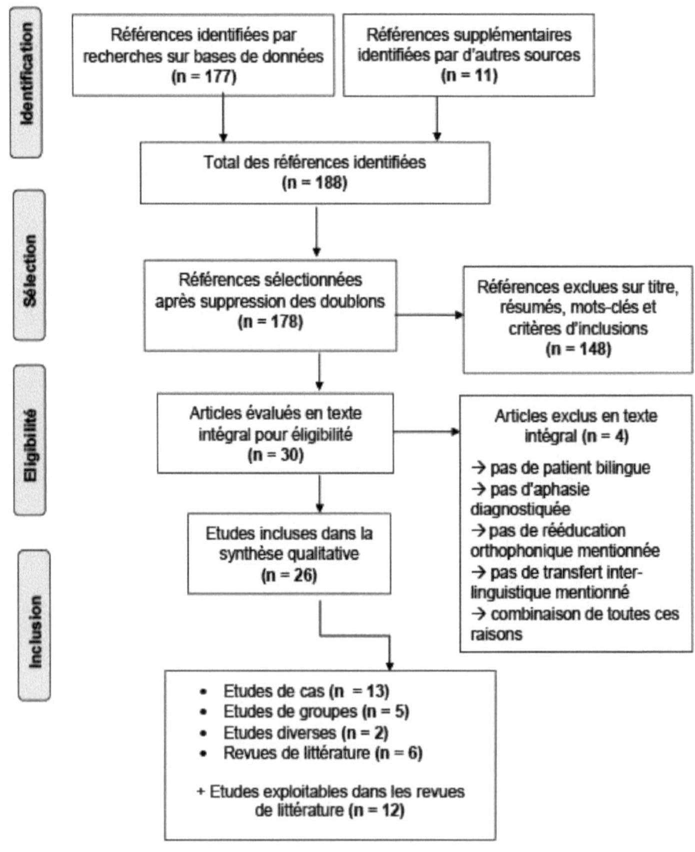

<u>APPENDIX I:</u> Studies used in literature reviews.

Type of study	Author(s)	Number of studies and date of publication	Number of studies excluded (exclusion criteria)	Number of studies selected
Literature review	*Ansaldo and Saidi, 2014.*	11 (1999-2002)	-studies already analysed individually: 6 -studies prior to 2000: 1 -study not recovered: 1	3
Literature review	*Faroqi-Shah, Frymark, Mullen, and Wang, 2010.*	13 (1980-2009)	-studies already analysed individually: 4 -studies prior to 2000: 4 -incomplete study (non exploitable): 1	4
Literature review	*Khachatryan, Vanhoof, Beyens, Goeleven, Thijs and Van Hulle, 2016.*	Number of studies and dates not specified.	-studies already analysed individually based on bibliography: 2 -studies prior to 2000: 14	1
Literature review	*Kohnert, 2009.*	12 (1975-2008)	-studies already analysed individually: 4 -studies prior to 2000: 4	4
Mini literature review	*Laganaro, 2014.*	10 (2001-2004)	-studies already analysed individually: 5 -studies prior to 2000: 0	5
Literature review	*Lorenzen and Muray, 2008.*	24 (1976-2006)*	-studies already analysed individually: 4 -studies prior to 2000: 9 -studies not taking into account the concept of generalisation: 7 -study not recovered: 1	3
Literature review	*Miller Amberber, 2011.*	41 (1914-2011)	-studies already analysed individually: 8 -studies prior to 2000 : 22 -study not recovered: 1	10

TOTAL eligible studies = 30

TOTAL usable studies after removing duplicates = 12

*In this review of the general literature (Lorenzen and Murray, 2008), only articles dealing with the rehabilitation of bilingual aphasics were taken into account.

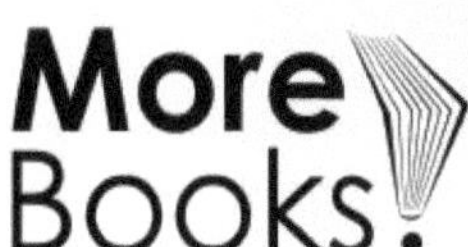

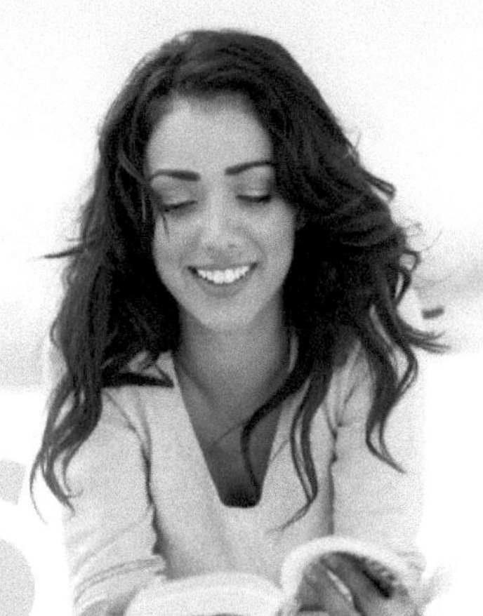

Buy your books fast and straightforward online - at one of world's fastest growing online book stores! Environmentally sound due to Print-on-Demand technologies.

Buy your books online at
www.morebooks.shop

Kaufen Sie Ihre Bücher schnell und unkompliziert online – auf einer der am schnellsten wachsenden Buchhandelsplattformen weltweit! Dank Print-On-Demand umwelt- und ressourcenschonend produzi ert.

Bücher schneller online kaufen
www.morebooks.shop

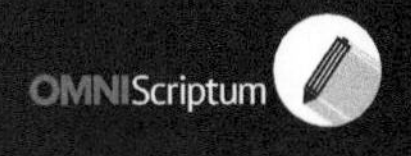

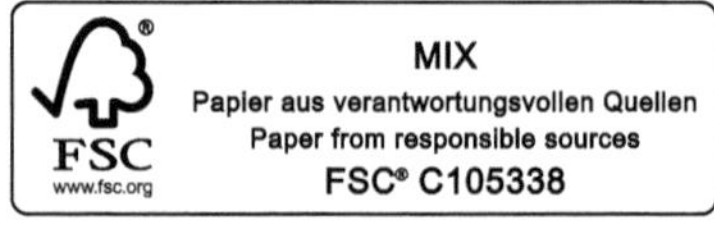

Printed by Books on Demand GmbH, Norderstedt / Germany